W9-AYQ-304

AGELESS YOGA

Rosie Reichmann

AGELESS YOGA

Astrolog ◆ The Quality of Life Series ◆

Series editor: Sara Bleich
Editor: Marion Duman
Cover design: Na'ama Yaffe
Layout and Graphics: Ruth Erez
Production Manager: Dan Gold
Photographs supplied by the author.

© Astrolog Publishing House 2001

ISBN 965-494-124-4

All rights reserved. No part of this publication may be reproduced,
stored in a retrieval system, or transmitted in any form or by any means,
electronic, mechanical, photocopying, recording or otherwise,
without the prior permission of the publisher.

Published by Astrolog Publishing House 2001

Astrolog Publishing House

P. O. Box 1123, Hod Hasharon 45111, Israel
Tel: 972-9-7412044
Fax: 972-9-7442714
E-Mail: info@astrolog.co.il

Printed in Israel

1 3 5 7 9 10 8 6 4 2

Contents

In loving memory of:

My parents, Avraham and Sarah Mendelowitz, of blessed memory, and my seven brothers and sisters who perished in the Holocaust.

My sister Helen, of blessed memory, whom I followed to England.

My husband and helpmeet, Peretz Reichmann, of blessed memory, who made all this possible.

My brothers Moshe and Arieh, of blessed memory, who more than anything symbolized the struggle for life.

Acknowledgments

I would like to express my heartfelt thanks and gratitude to:

My pupil Fran Naim, who spent many days patiently and accurately collating and editing every detail, and by whose initiative and energy this book has been published,

Pazit Naim who, thanks to Fran's inspiration, succeeded in bringing the words, positions, and feelings to life in her special photographs.

My neighbor Yehudit Vigdor for her professional suggestions.

Ofra Hazan for the translation of one of my lectures.

To all my pupils throughout the years who had faith in me and helped me develop the tool that gave me life.

And especially to my niece, Miriam Shenar, for everything she does for me, as well as for her help with this book - all my love and appreciation, from the bottom of my heart.

(Rivka)
Rosie Reichmann

One of Rosie's lectures on yoga

Yoga is nature's special way of maintaining physical and mental health. It is a technique of self-discipline that can be practiced at any age.

Yoga is an ancient health art that was developed and perfected over hundreds of years in India, and was acknowledged worldwide as the best way to keep the body and the mind healthy and young by means of exercise. It helps all of our muscles, bones and internal organs operate at the peak of efficiency. It has an astonishing power to refresh and calm the nerves and the mind, and to grant inner strength and energy.

This is part of the charm of yoga. If you want a full life, filled with energy, start practicing yoga. You will be surprised at the change in your health.

Presumably, you cope with many problems, your day is too short, and you are under constant pressure. It is reasonable to assume that you do your work sitting down; you spend most of the day seated, hardly moving a muscle. Life makes endless demands on your physical and emotional resources. It is possible that you like your lifestyle, but occasionally things mount up and "suffocate" you.

Unexpected complications, disappointments, errors, misunderstandings, nervousness, and minor or major crises occur. These things can cause an ulcer, for example. Most people are unable to control their emotions, and are hurt as a result.

This is where yoga can be of tremendous help. It is a tool that will help you discard all your fears. You will learn how to gain release and freedom of thought. You will reshape yourself. You will acquire a more serene outlook on life, and you will be more productive in every field. For instance, you will learn correct breathing, which is the essence of life.

Deep breathing is known to calm the nervous system. It also reduces tension and improves concentration. Oxygen is the only thing we cannot live without. If need be, we can exist without food for up to a month and without water for a few days. But without the breathing that is so precious to us, we cannot exist for more than a few minutes. Having said that, few people know how to breathe correctly.

There is a little tale about the senses arguing about which of them is the most important. The senses under discussion are the ones that are recognized in yoga: Sight, Hearing, Thought, and Breathing.

In order to prove its importance, Sight leaves a particular person's eyes. A year later, it returns, and asks the person: "Well, how's life without me?" The answer was: "Like a man who cannot see."

Afterwards, Hearing leaves. A year later, it returns and asks the same question. The answer was: "Nothing disturbed me, and I enjoyed the silence that surrounded me."

When Thought left and returned a year later, the answer was: "I was like a fool for a year."

Then it was Breathing's turn. All the senses shouted: "Please don't leave! Without you, we can't survive!"

And they declared breathing to be queen of the senses.

Stories aside, we do not pay attention to the way we use our breathing. Yoga teaches us how to improve our health by means of correct breathing. We breathe 23,000 times a day; it is the first and last thing we do in this world. But how frequently do we stop to examine our breathing and try to breathe more deeply, more slowly and more calmly?

Of all the yoga exercises, the breathing exercises require the least effort. In fact, they must be performed effortlessly.

They take up very little time and can be done while sitting, lying down, or walking.

Countless books have been written about yoga, especially hata yoga, the most popular current. Hatha yoga focuses on physical health alongside the influence on thought. Raja yoga focuses on the rational processes that are meant to control the body. Jenana yoga is the yoga of knowing the I - the person's essence.

Yoga practice and study are a lifelong occupation. When we engage in it, we discover that it is full of great wisdom. Compare it to the study of the Talmud. Yoga deals with everything to do with health: diet, posture, breathing, eating habits, relaxation, walking, thinking, sitting, sleeping, and even getting out of bed.

The aim of hatha yoga is to make us aware of our body and to bring it under full control. Its practice can be divided into three parts: control of thought, of the body, and of breathing. The three must be practiced together. With practice, the person acquires self-control. This is a great achievement. Moreover, by practicing the yoga movements, we improve the flexibility of our body.

The first step is to rid ourselves of all emotions of fear. Contemplate the future with confidence, faith, joy, patience, and determination. Control your emotions. Foster a positive outlook on life, one that will give you health and energy. Remember - you can do anything you want, provided that you have will power. Negative thoughts destroy and age people. Worry is at the top of the list. It is followed by tension, anger, nervousness, gloom, sadness, self-pity, habitual late nights, a lack of physical exercise, overeating, and weight that goes up and down like a yo-yo. Those are the principal negative foundations that must be avoided.

Everything in life is habit. You can achieve wonderful things with good habits, but you can ruin good health with bad habits. For instance, eating when you are emotionally hurt or overtired is bad for you. You should always rest before eating, and it is important to ensure that the people eating with you are also relaxed.

The best way to relax during the day is by deep breathing - always, of course, through the nose. Practice deep breathing every time you are outside in the fresh air. It will give you lust for life and it will calm you down - temporarily. Go walking every time you have free time. That is a law of nature. Hatha yoga teaches that work is a blessing, but don't "bless" yourself from morning to night!

Sleep on a hard mattress. Clean out your intestines. Eat unpeeled fruit and vegetables. Eat slowly. Don't use white sugar; use brown sugar instead - or, better still, honey. Replace table salt with sea salt. Drink a lot of water between meals. Don't drown your food with liquid. Eating and drinking together is a bad habit. Avoid drinking beverages that are too hot or too cold. Use a lot of polyunsaturated, cold pressed oil in your salads. This will prevent your bones from becoming brittle and fragile at a later stage in life. Walk and sit up straight.

Being healthy is something you owe yourself. Don't feel guilty if you prepare something special for yourself to eat even though the people around you don't like it. Relax whenever you can devote a few moments to it. Practice yoga and watch your figure all your life. Nurture inner quiet, truth, honesty, and simplicity. Those are a few of the basic rules of hatha yoga.

You can destroy yourself by constant worry, or you can be full of life and happiness. Everything is in your head. We can add years to our lives and, in addition, preserve our quality of life - in other words, add years to our life and life to our years. You don't get old just because the calendar says so. There are people who have always looked old and others who always look young. It is a matter of outlook on life.

Make your body live by daily practice. Don't neglect it and say, "I do enough every day." Chores and housework have no effect on your body. In contrast, yoga rectifies your posture, strengthens your neglected muscles, and repairs those that have atrophied. There is no part of your body that does not benefit greatly from practicing yoga. The body becomes younger despite the fact that the person is aging.

Relax as much as you can, relax while driving, sitting, walking, cooking. You don't have to lie down in order to relax. Having said that, it is very effective to lie on the floor once a day, preferably in the afternoon, and relax every muscle in your body. Fifteen minutes of this daily routine will be of tremendous benefit to you.

Eat the correct food slowly. Remember that proteins are your friends and carbohydrates are your enemies. It would seem that the enemy has a great hold on us: we all know that we must not indulge in empty calories - they ruin the figure and cause us to suffer later simply for the sake of five minutes of enjoying unsuitable food. It shows that we must improve our self-discipline. There is no reason to become fat as we get older. The body must be a source of pride throughout our lives. Avoid what is called "the middle-age spread." When people stop doing the activities they did when they were young - running, jumping, skipping, swimming - they begin to gain weight. They substitute food for other pleasures they no longer experience. They eat more they need and do less exercise than they need. Eat when you are hungry. Don't watch the clock. Don't eat calorie-rich foods. Don't eat too much at one meal.

In ancient Egypt, it is said, the royal palaces employed a physician to check the health and the eating habits of the rulers by means of interrogating the chefs in the kitchens. If the answer to the question, "How do you feed the king?" was: "He only eats when he's hungry," the physician would leave quickly, realizing that there was nothing for him to do there. If he was told in another noble house that the head of the household insisted on eating raw fruit and vegetables (more than cooked ones), he would also leave quickly, knowing that he was not needed there. However, when he went into a kitchen in which rich foods were being prepared, he smiled and embraced the chef. "Half of what he eats here keeps him alive," he remarked. "The other half keeps us - the physicians - alive."

We must keep away from the physician as much as possible. It is our duty to be healthy. We must make the effort to cultivate good habits instead of bad ones that compel us to invent endless excuses. Don't use your car when you can walk. Use your body. Don't just push buttons. Don't lie in the sun until your body is burned just to impress those around you. Nothing ages the skin more than the sun.

Hatha yoga is not about doing acrobatics, it is not competitive. It is an individual matter. The pupil gets out of it what he puts into it. Every movement has an aim. Practicing yoga requires understanding in order to derive the maximum benefit and enjoyment from it. It is a method that was developed carefully, based on an acute understanding of the human body and its functions. It works to prevent the degeneration of the body with age.

If you want something that is beyond your reach, you will be unsatisfied. Avoid craving and envy. They are generally accompanied by bitterness and anger. The path to happiness lies in self-control and in unselfish giving to those who are less fortunate. Controlling our emotions can spare us negative, destructive thoughts such as anger, resentment, hatred, fear, worry, and envy. All of those destroy happiness. Keep your sense of humor and smile. It's difficult to worry when you're smiling. Build a happy personality for yourself, be creative. Direct yourself toward a positive purpose. Be hopeful. Believe in yourself; you can be your own best friend, or your own worst enemy. The choice is yours.

The secret of good health and satisfaction is to know yourself. Know your body and how to take care of it. There is an enormous difference between the blessings of money and health. Money is the thing that people want most, but enjoy least. Health is the thing that people enjoy most, but envy each other for least. Health is the supreme blessing.

The poorest man will not give up his health for money, while the rich man will gladly give up his money for good health.

Yoga does not pretend to be a cure-all, but rather a preventive measure that teaches us to protect and improve ourselves before it's too late.

Be healthy instead of "get well."

Stop worrying about what other people have and you don't. You won't be happier when you have it. Avoid cravings like that because they destroy satisfaction and happiness. If you want nothing, it means that you have everything you want, and you are truly happy. A great philosopher once defined happiness as wanting what you have, not what you do not have.

Yoga is a kind of self-development in every sphere of life. It is an awareness that leads to a fuller life for those who are prepared to contribute to, think about, and act for their own benefit. The rewards are health, vitality, and peace of mind. The West should be grateful to the East for the gift of yoga, which is a very rewarding way of life.

Resume
My personal journey to yoga

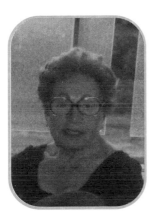 I was born in 1917 in the village of Giraltovce in Czechoslovakia, the fourth of twelve children.

I always remember my childhood as extremely happy, and I was influenced by the love and optimism I observed between my parents, and by the simplicity that epitomized our lives at that time.

I reached England in 1937, and that period is characterized not only by the World War (and the blitz), but also by the fight for survival and existence as an immigrant in the relatively closed British society.

Youthful dreams remained unattainable then - until the long journey to yoga.

The change started with a bad movement that led to a severe pain in my back and insomnia for 20 years.

The focus of my life at the time was on finding a cure from the best physicians in England and Switzerland - to no avail. I reached the "Iyengar" center in London at age 40, and became aware of the fact that there is no age at which a person cannot help himself. I learned that by means of positive thinking, optimism, and faith, it is possible to achieve.

I overcame the intolerable pain that had been my constant companion for years, and at the end of four years of intensive study, I became a teacher. I took my first steps with a group of women at the neighborhood synagogue in London.

For the last 25 years, I have been living in Israel, and teaching young and old women every day. I believe that yoga is also a mission; what helped me can help others.

Introduction to the exercises

Exercise according to the yoga method helps the body in every possible condition, but the best way to start yoga is when the body is healthy and balanced.

It is important to exercise once a day or at least once or twice a week.

The body must be introduced gradually to yoga practice: initially, the session should take about a quarter hour, little by little getting longer until it reaches one hour a day.

Yoga should be practiced at a fixed time. Each person determines the time that suits him during the day - whether it is first thing in the morning or after work in the evening.

Occasionally, during yoga practice, we may feel pains in various parts of our body. There is no need to worry: this may be blockages in the body being released. Through Iyengar yoga, we become familiar with our body, even though this may sometimes be painful. In time, if we persist, renewed vitality begins to flow through our body.

- The yoga method is good for people of any age.
- It is important to practice it at least once every two days.
- Perseverance yields results.

Preparing for yoga practice

We exercise barefoot (summer or winter).

Long hair is tied back.

All jewelry is removed beforehand.

Fixed instructions for yoga

1. Remember to relax the body before every exercise!

2. Remember to inhale deeply through your nose at the beginning of the exercise. You also exhale through your nose.

3. Each time you bend or straighten up, do so gradually, vertebra by vertebra.

4. Each time you stand up after lying down, this is how you do it: Turn over on your side in a fetal position, and push your body up very slowly with your arms.

Breathing in yoga

Every movement in yoga is accompanied by deep breaths.

> At the beginning of every movement, inhale; toward the end of the movement, exhale.

This is how we breathe in yoga:

Inhale deeply through your nose at the beginning of every movement.
Exhale an emptying breath, also through your nose, toward the end of the movement.
When we inhale, we let clean air enter our lungs.
When we exhale, we get rid of the air that is not good for our body.
The more we fill our lungs to capacity, and the more we empty them completely, the more we improve our health.

Abdominal breathing

- Inhale as much air as possible through your nose, and try to ensure that your stomach swells up during inhalation.
- Hold the air in your lungs for a few seconds.
- Exhale it completely through your nose; while exhaling, contract your abdomen, which moves toward your back.
- When inhaling and exhaling, try not to move your chest and shoulders.

Several ways of performing yoga exercises

There are various ways to perform yoga exercises. Some exercises can be done sitting or standing, sitting on a chair or on a mattress, and so on. There are six main methods:

- Standing, with chairs;

- Seated, with chairs;

- Sitting on a carpet or mattress;

- Lying on a carpet or mattress;

- Standing on one's shoulders - the queen of yoga;

- Standing on one's head - the king of yoga.

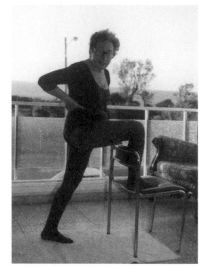

Each person chooses the type of exercise that suits him. The most highly recommended exercise is movement in conjunction with chairs, because it is the most effective - it requires less effort than other exercises, and it is very beneficial to the body:

> **More powerful with less effort**

- The yoga method employed here is "hatha yoga."

- The welcome effect of hatha yoga exercises on the body lasts up to 12 hours after the session, while practice with chairs has a beneficial effect on the body for 24 hours.

- We exercise every day or every other day.

- It is a good idea to select the type of activity before beginning to exercise: for example, exercising with chairs, standing, and then seated; or standing exercises and then sitting on the mattress.

Exercises standing up

Positions for starting the exercises

Standing

There are six basic standing positions:

- Standing up straight with legs close together.

- Standing up straight (with legs 10 cm apart).

- Standing with legs slightly apart.

    Standing with legs wide apart (facing forward, your face in the center of your body)

- Standing in a triangle (a) = step position, legs apart, right leg and body facing to the right. Both legs are straight and taut.

- Standing in a triangle (b) = step position, legs apart, right leg and body facing to the right. The front leg is bent and the back leg is straight and taut.

Warm-up exercise

The warm-up exercise is the exercise that precedes every activity in yoga.

Breathing: both inhalation and exhalation are performed through the nose.

- Stand erect with legs close together.

- Your hands are at your sides.

Remember to inhale deeply through your nose at the beginning of the exercise.

- Stretch your arms (inhale deeply) upward and forward.

- Both your hands face forward.

- Bring your arms back to your sides in the same way they were raised (exhale).

Do this twice.

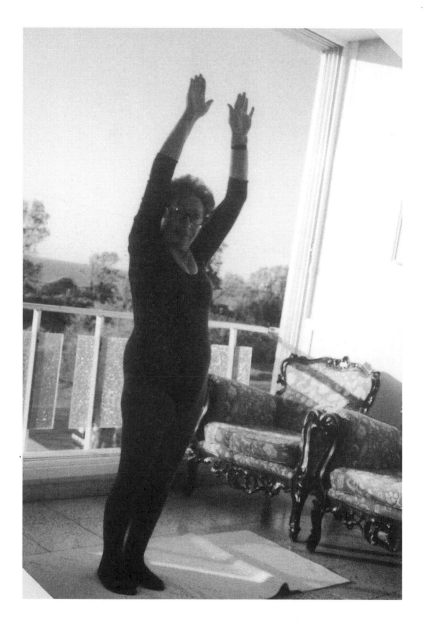

- Lift up your arms and inhale.

- Bend your knees slightly, and stretch your arms forward, as in the previous movement (exhale).

Remain in this position for the count of three.

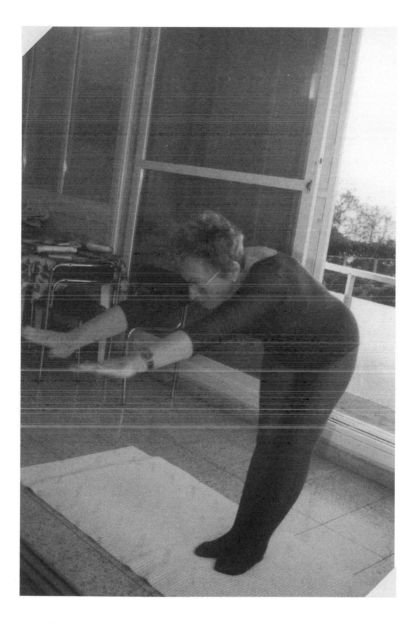

- Stretch your arms upward again (inhale). This time, the backs of your hands face each other.

- Move your arms outward at shoulder height, and bend the upper part of your body forward (exhale).

- Bend your knees, release your arms, your back still leaning forward. Swing both arms forward and backward at your sides.

- Swing your arms, crossing them in front; alternate between your right arm being nearer to your body and then your left arm being nearer to it - a kind of scissor movement in front of your body.

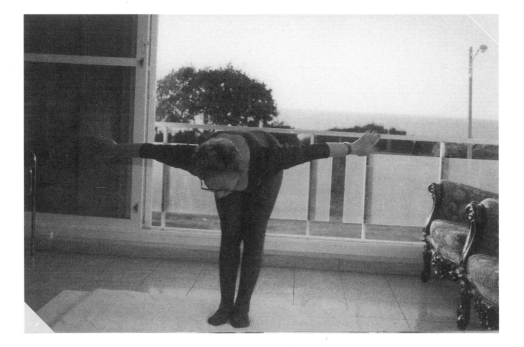

Making the waist and the center of the back more pliant

- Stand up straight or with legs slightly apart, arms at your sides.
- Raise your right shoulder to your right ear, without moving your head. Then raise your left shoulder to your left ear.

Do this exercise five times on each side.

- Place your hands in your armpits (inhale).
  Your right hand is in your right armpit and your left hand is in your left armpit.
- Raise your elbows.
- Twist your body backward to the right.

Remain in this position for a few seconds (exhale).

Now do this movement to the left.

Do this exercise three times.

Between exercises, relax your body.

Making the waist pliant (continued)

- Stand with your legs further apart (exhale).
- Place your right arm behind your back. The back of your right hand touches the back of your left hip. Place your left hand on your right shoulder.
- Twist around in the direction of the right shoulder (inhale).

Remain in this position for a few seconds.

Repeat the exercise for the left side:

Right hand on left shoulder and turning to the left.

Do this exercise five times.

Making the body pliant

- Relax your body.

- All the muscles are relaxed.

- Place your hands behind your back on your kidneys, that is, upward from the waist.

This is the finger position: The thumbs face forward, and the fingertips face backward, touching one another.

- While inhaling, turn your right knee and your right shoulder inward toward the left. Turn your head to the left as well.

- Straighten your knee and shoulder, and turn your head to face forward again (exhale).

Do this exercise three to five times.

Repeat the movements in the opposite direction:

- While inhaling, turn your left knee and your left shoulder inward toward the right.
  Turn your head to the right as well.

- Straighten your knee and shoulder, and turn your head to face forward again (exhale).

Do this exercise three to five times.

Releasing the shoulder-blades (stage 1)

- Stand with your legs slightly apart, arms at your sides, and your chin resting on your chest.

- Slowly raise your head, looking straight ahead.

- Raise your shoulders while inhaling.

- Bring your shoulder-blades closer together by squeezing (exhale).

- Raise your chin. Your shoulders are still raised.

- Relax.

- Rest your chin on your chest once again. Bend your knees (inhale).

- Lean the upper part of your body forward and down.

- Place your hands on your feet for a little while (exhale).

- Straighten your legs. In this exercise, you feel your calf muscles.

- Slowly straighten your back and your knees (inhale).

- Place your hands behind your head, above the back of your neck.

- Gently straighten your head and release (exhale).

Do this exercise three times.

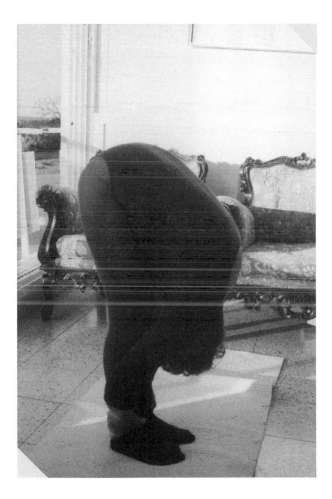

Releasing the shoulder-blades (stage 2)

- Stand with your legs slightly apart, arms hanging at your sides, your chin touching your chest.

- Raise your head, facing forward.

- Raise your shoulders while inhaling.

- Squeeze the two shoulder-blades together backward while exhaling.

Remain in this position for the count of three.

- Once again, stretch your arms upward.
  This time, the backs of your hands face each other (inhale).

- Raise your arms straight out at your sides at shoulder height, and at the same time bend forward (exhaling).

- Bend your knees, release your arms, and swing them together backward and forward at the sides of your body.

- Swing your arms, crossing them in front; alternate between your right arm being nearer to your body and then your left arm being nearer to it (scissors).

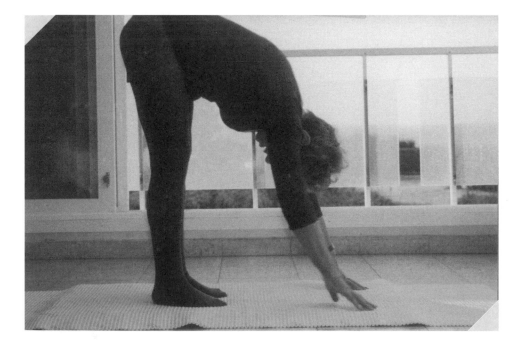

Releasing the abdominal muscles

- Stand with your legs apart, your feet in line with your shoulders.
- Place your fingers on your clavicle (inhale).
- Put your knees together and contract your thighs.
- While doing so, pull your abdomen in (exhale).
- Bend over.
  Your elbows touch your knees (or come close to them).
- Straighten up and relax your muscles while exhaling.

Do this exercise five times.

Stretching the tendons of the legs and making them pliant

This is a good exercise for the knees and for the sciatic nerve.

- Stand up straight, hands on your hips.
- Feet together.
- Inhale and move your bent right leg behind your left leg, which bends slightly.
- Move your right leg (from the pelvis) forward next to the left leg.
- The toes of your right foot touch the floor (exhale).

Bend your knees slowly about five times (inhale).

- Stretch your right leg backward (exhale).

Bend down 10 times.

This is how you bend down:

- Bend your front knee, with the heel of your back leg stretched as taut as possible.
- Pull your body lightly downward 10 times. (This can be quickly or slowly.)

Do this exercise twice with each leg.

Relaxing the legs

- Release your legs and stretch them.

Stretch and relax your legs alternately several times.

Releasing the back of the neck and stretching the body

This exercise requires effort and perseverance in order to obtain results.

- Stand with your legs wide apart, head facing forward.
- Bend over and move your right elbow close to your inner right thigh.
- Place your right arm below the right knee or thigh in front of the body.
- Place your left hand behind you on your buttocks, and let your hands come close to each other or clasp each other (if possible).
- In this position, bend your right knee and straighten it, alternately.
- During the exercise, your head is turned to the left and upward.
- Remain in this position for the count of three each time.

Do 10 of these bends.

Repeat the exercise on the other side:

- Bend over and move your left elbow close to your inner left thigh.
- Place your left arm below the left knee or thigh in front of the body.
- Place your right hand behind you on your buttocks, and let your hands come close to each other or clasp each other (if possible).
- In this position, bend your left knee and straighten it, alternately.
- During the exercise, your head is turned to the right and upward.
- Remain in this position for the count of three each time.

Do 10 of these bends.

Stretching the side of the body

- Stand in step position to the right (inhale).
- Stretch your right arm out to the right (the one that's on the side of the front knee).
- Pull your stretched arm toward the ceiling, as if pushing the ceiling (exhale). The arm moves from the front of the body directly upward, keeping it straight.
- Return your arm to its original position.
- Remain in this position for the count of five.

Do this exercise three to five times.

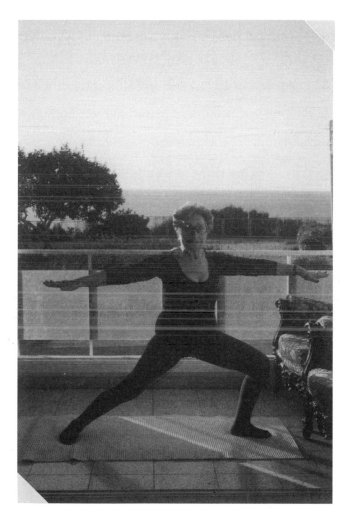

Repeat the exercise in the other direction:

- Stand in step position to the left (inhale).
- Stretch your left arm out to the left (the hand that's on the side of the front knee).
- Pull your stretched arm toward the ceiling, as if pushing the ceiling (exhale). The arm moves from the front of the body directly upward, keeping it straight.
- Return your arm to its original position.
- Remain in this position for the count of five.

Do this exercise three to five times.

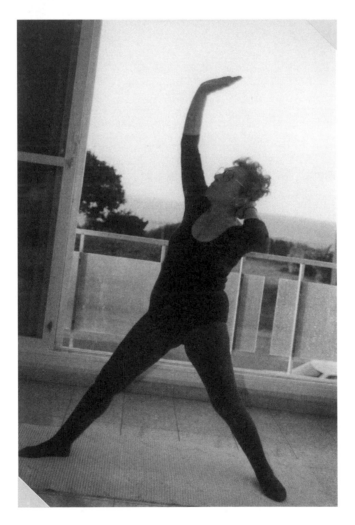

Hip turns

- Stand with your legs slightly apart (inhale).
- Stretch your arms out in front of you, and then upward, with a 30-cm gap between them.
- Your inner palms face forward.
- Slowly swing your arms to the right and downward until they touch the floor, and then to the left and upward - in a circle.
  The movement is performed in large circles from the waist; the entire upper part of the body takes part in it.

Do the circular movement of the arms five times to the right and five times to the left.

Strengthening the inner thighs

- Stand with your legs wide apart.
- Lift and stretch your arms forward and upward while inhaling.
- Bend forward from your waist, exhaling. Relax your hands and release the muscles.
- Each hand holds the toes of the corresponding foot between the thumb and index finger (right hand holds right foot, left hand holds left foot).
- Bend your right knee to the right, simultaneously straightening and stretching the left leg.
- Continue the movement immediately: Straighten and stretch the right knee, and bend the left one.

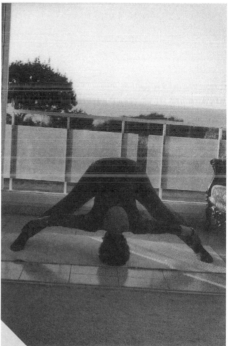

Do this exercise five times with each leg.

Releasing the lower back

- Stand with your legs apart, your knees slightly bent (inhale).
- Place your hands on your thighs.
- Bend forward slowly, and then gradually straighten up, vertebra by vertebra, while exhaling.

Do this exercise three times.

Stretching the back of the neck and releasing it

- Stand up straight with your legs together or sit straight up on a chair (inhale).
- Place your hands behind your head, above the back of the neck, thumbs next to the ears, fingertips touching. Your hands serve as a lever for pulling the head upward.
- Pull your head upward, and then slowly release, exhaling gently.

Do this exercise three times in a completely relaxed way.

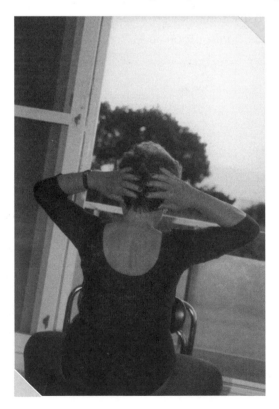

Stretching the tendons and muscles of the legs and releasing them

- Stand in step position to the right.
- Place your hands on the floor on either side of your right foot.

Do 10 bends.

- Breathe as necessary.
- Afterwards, move your body slightly backward while exhaling.
  This is how your move your body:
  Your right leg stretches and straightens, and you raise your toes.
  At the same time, lower your left heel (the back one) to the floor, and
  slowly relcasc (likc a foot sccsaw).

Rock your entire taut body 10 times gently back and forth.

Do this exercise three times.

Repeat the exercise with the left foot:

- Stand in step position to the left.
- Place your hands on the floor on either side of your left foot.

Do 10 bends.

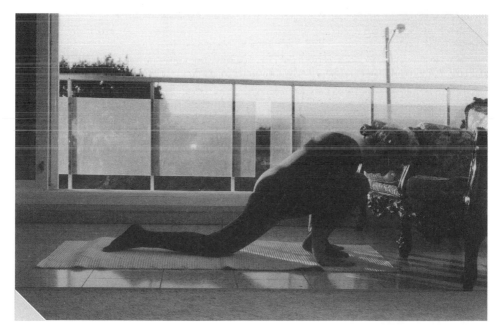

- Breathe as necessary.

- Afterwards, move your body slightly backward while exhaling.
  This is how your move your body:
  Your left leg stretches and straightens, and you raise your toes.
  At the same time, lower your right heel (the back one) to the floor, and
  slowly release (like a foot seesaw).

Rock your whole taut body 10 times gently back and forth.

Do this exercise three times.

Triangle exercises

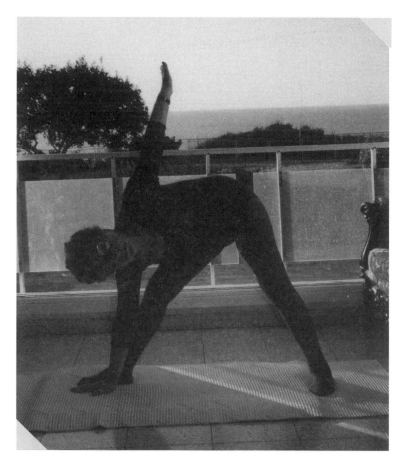

Releasing the body with triangle exercises

The exercise is good for the neck and the back of the neck.

- Stand in wide step position to the right, your legs taut and straight, your arms at your sides.
- Lift your straight right arm to shoulder height while inhaling.
- Bend to the right and place your right hand on your right foot (exhale).
- Move your stretched left arm to the right, in the direction of your right hand (which is resting on your right foot).
- Remain in the position for the count of 10.
- Place your left hand on your waist, behind your back (inhale).
- Move your right hand to your outer left ankle.
- While turning the upper part of your body, look to the left and upward (exhale).
- Remain in this position for the count of 10.

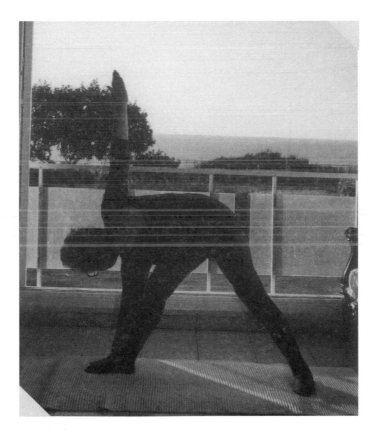

Repeat the exercise on the left side:

- Stand in wide step position to the left, your legs taut and straight, your arms at your sides.
- Lift your straight left arm to shoulder height while inhaling.
- Bend to the left and place your left hand on your left foot (exhale).
- Move your stretched right arm to the left, in the direction of your left hand (which is resting on your left foot).
- Remain in the position for the count of 10.
- Place your right hand on your hip, behind your back (inhale).
- Move your left hand to your outer right ankle.
- While turning the upper part of your body, look to the right and upward (exhale).
- Remain in this position for the count of 10.

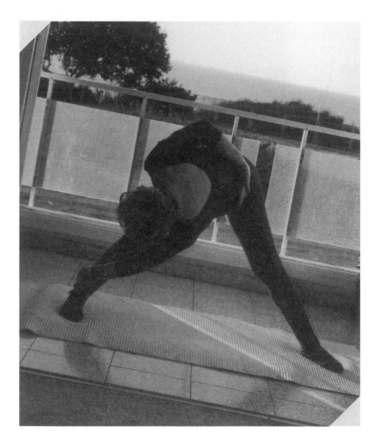

Triangle exercises for releasing the entire body

- Spread your legs further apart, your arms hanging at your sides.
- Bend your right knee to the side and turn your body to the right.
- Stand in a step position to the right and left, alternately.
- Lift your arms to shoulder height (inhale).
- When you stand in step position to the right, your left hand is stretched forward to the right, and your right arm goes backward (the back of your right arm faces the floor).
- Both arms are at shoulder height while doing the exercise.
- Turn the upper part of your body to the left. Your right arm pulls to the side and your left arm pulls backward (exhale).
- Stand in a wide step position to the right, your legs taut and straight, your arms at your sides.
- Lift your straight right arm to shoulder height while inhaling.
- Bend to the right and place your right hand on your right foot (exhale).
- Move your stretched left arm to the right, in the direction of your right hand (which is resting on your right foot).
- Remain in this position for the count of 10.

- Place your left hand on your waist, behind your back (inhale).
- Move your right hand to your outer left ankle.
- While turning the upper part of your body, look to the left and upward (exhale).
- Remain in this position for the count of 10.
- Move your right hand to your other foot while turning the upper part of your body.
- Move your left hand to your waist behind your back (exhale).
- Straighten up.

- Bend your left knee forward, and turn your body to the left in step position.
- Lift your arms (inhale), and stretch them at shoulder height, each arm in the direction of the corresponding foot.
- Touch the floor with your left hand next to your bent left leg.
- The upper part of your body leans forward and sideways to the left.
- Stretch your left arm forward, slightly twisting the upper part of your body.
- Remain in this position for the count of 10.

- Move your left hand to your right foot, slightly twisting the upper part of your body.
- Move your right hand to your waist behind your back.

Do each exercise twice.

Repeat the exercise with the other foot:

- Stand in a wide step position to the left, your legs taut and straight, your arms at your sides.
- Lift your straight left arm to shoulder height while inhaling.
- Bend to the left and place your left hand on your left foot (exhale).
- Move your straight right arm to the left, in the direction of your left hand (which is resting on your left foot).
- Remain in this position for the count of 10.
- Place your right hand on your waist, behind your back (inhale).
- Move your left hand to your outer right ankle.
- While turning the upper part of your body, look to the right and upward (exhale).
- Remain in this position for the count of 10.

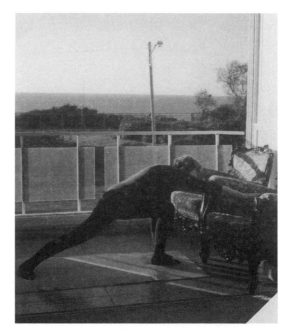

Continuation of the triangle exercises for making the body pliant

- Relax your body.
- Stand in step position to the right, your legs wide apart, your body turned to the right, your legs straight and taut.
- Inhale deeply.
- The upper part of your body is turned to the right.
- Slowly and gently slide your right hand along your right leg until it touches the floor in front of your right foot (exhale).
- Your legs are straight throughout the exercise.
- Remain in this stretch for a few seconds and slowly straighten up.

Repeat the exercise with the left leg:

- Inhale deeply.
- The upper part of your body is turned to the left.
- Slowly and gently slide your left hand along your left leg until it touches the floor in front of the left foot (exhale).
- Your legs are straight throughout the exercise.
- Remain in this stretch for a few seconds and slowly straighten up.

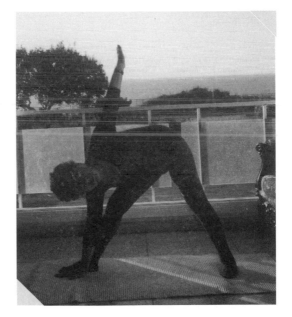

Strengthening the spine and the inner thighs

Stage 1

- Stand with your legs wide apart, facing forward (inhale).

- Bend your body forward at the waist.

- Grasp your two big toes between your thumbs and two fingers - each hand grasps a foot.

- Bend to the right, bending your right knee and your right elbow together. Your whole left side is stretched.

- Remain in this position for the count of 10.

- Continue to the left side, bending your left knee and your left elbow together, and stretching your whole right side.

- Remain in this position for the count of 10.

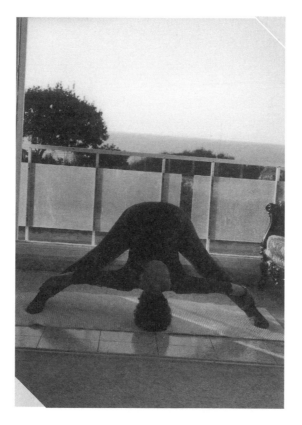

Stage 2

- Hold your ankles in your hands: your right hand holds your right ankle, and your left hand holds your left ankle.
- Lift your head, inhale, and lower your head toward the floor, exhaling. You can feel the inner part of your thighs being stretched.
- Lift your head again (inhale).
- Bend the upper part of your body forward and downward.
- Place your elbows and forearms on the floor. Lift yourself up on your toes.
- Lower your head (exhale).
- Straighten up vertebra by vertebra.
- Straighten up very slowly.
- Turn your toes inward, opposite one another.
- Stand on your tocs, and turn your heels to face each other.
- In this way, you zigzag your feet inward until they are slightly apart.
- Relax your body.

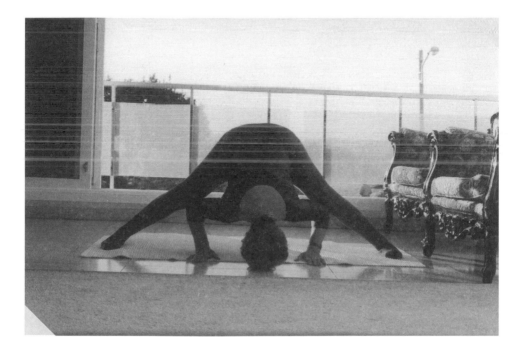

Treating the back - backward stretch

- Stand in step position to the right.
- Fold your arms behind your back, the back of your hands facing upward.
- Turn the upper part of your body to the right (inhale).
- Bend in the direction of your right foot; now the back of your hand is facing the floor.
- Lift your arms toward the ceiling.
- In this position, place your chest on your right thigh, your nose on your right knee.
- Your hands do not change their position (exhale).
- Straighten up and relax.

Do this exercise three times to the right.

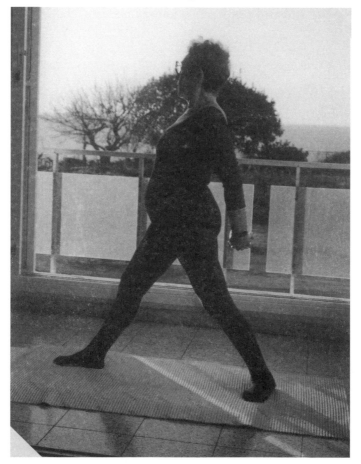

Repeat the exercise on the left side:

- Fold your arms behind your back, the back of your hands facing upward.
- Turn the upper part of your body to the left, and change the direction of the fingers. Now the back of your hand is facing the floor.
- Bend in the direction of your left foot and lift your arms toward the ceiling.
- In this position, place your chest on your left thigh, your nose on your left knee.
- Straighten up and relax.

Do this exercise three times to the left.

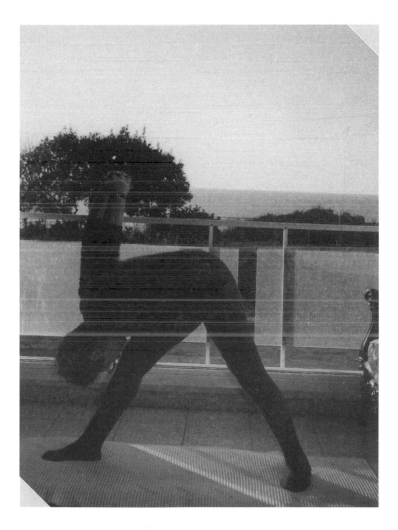

Improving circulation (Releasing the shoulder and thigh joints)

Limb turns

- Stand up straight.

- Place your right hand on your hip.

- Your left arm and your right leg perform the movement.

- Turn your left arm (from the shoulder joint) and your bent right leg (from the thigh joint) in large, slow turns, alternately, first backward and then forward.

Make six turns in each direction.

Repeat the exercise on the other side:

- Place your left hand on your hip.

- Your right arm and your left leg perform the movement.

- Turn your right arm (from the shoulder joint) and your bent left leg (from the thigh joint) in large, slow turns, alternately, first backward and then forward.

Make six turns in each direction.

Releasing the buttocks

Stage 1 - Warming the area

- Stand with your legs slightly apart.

- Place your hands on your hips.

- Move your pelvis, while standing, in large circular movements first to the right, forward, left and to the back, and then the opposite, over and over, a flowing turn of the whole pelvis (like a belly dancer).

Do the movement five times to the right and five times to the left.

Stage 2 - Hip turns

- Stand with your legs slightly apart.

- Place your hands on your hips.

- Bend the upper part of your body to the right and backward, continuing to the left, and returning to the middle.

- The movement is a flowing circular movement.

Do the movement five times to the right and five times to the left.

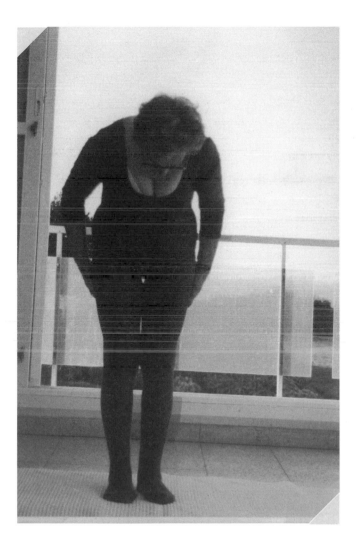

Treating the abdominal and back muscles

Stage 1 - Contracting and relaxing

- Stand with your legs slightly apart.
- Place both hands on your back, in the kidney region above your waistline (inhale).
- Push your hands on your back while contracting your abdominal muscles inward.
  There is pressure from the direction of the abdominal muscles toward the back and pressure of the hands and of the back toward the abdomen.
- Bend your knees slightly.
  Don't lock them.
- Exhale and straighten up.

Stage 2 - Flexibility

- Stand with your legs slightly apart.
- Your hands are still on your back above the waistline (inhale).
- Your elbows and shoulders turn to the right and backward (exhale).
- Inhale while your elbows and shoulders turn to the left and backward (exhale).

Do this exercise five times on each side.

Stage 3 - Flexibility

- Stand with your legs slightly apart (inhale).
- Place your hands on your hips.
- Bend to the right - the bend comes from the right hip (exhale).
- Remain in this position for a few seconds.

Repeat the bend six times.

- Stand with your legs slightly apart (inhale).
- Place your hands on your hips.
- Bend to the left - the bend comes from the left hip (exhale).
- Remain in this position for a few seconds.

Repeat the bend six times.

Treating the muscles of the front of the body and the back

- Stand with your legs slightly apart.
- Place your hands behind your head.
- Your elbows face forward at the sides of your temples (inhale).
- Gently bend forward (knees bent or locked) until your elbows touch your knees or at least come close to them (exhale).
- Move your knees slightly apart, and continue to bend in the direction of the floor, your elbows pulling toward the floor.
- Straighten your knees.
- Straighten up slowly, vertebra by vertebra.
- Your head straightens up last (inhale).
- Stand up straight (exhale).

Stretching the body

- Stand with your legs wide apart (step position to the right). Inhale.
- Stretch your right arm out to the right.
- Turn your left arm backward (exhale).
- Remain in the stretch position for the count of 10.
- Place your right hand on the floor next to the outside of the right foot.
- Hold out your left foot forward in the direction of the right leg (inhale).
- Remain in this position for the count of 10 (exhale).
- Place your left hand on the back of your neck.
- Lift your right arm and stretch to the right (inhale).
- Bend your right knee.
- Your right elbow touches your left knee (exhale).
- Remain in this position for the count of 10.
- Straighten up (inhale).

- Move your right hand to your left ankle by turning your hip.

- Move your bent left arm behind your back (exhale).

- The back of your hand rests on your right hip.

- Remain in this position for the count of 10.

- Straighten up.

Repeat this movement twice on the right.

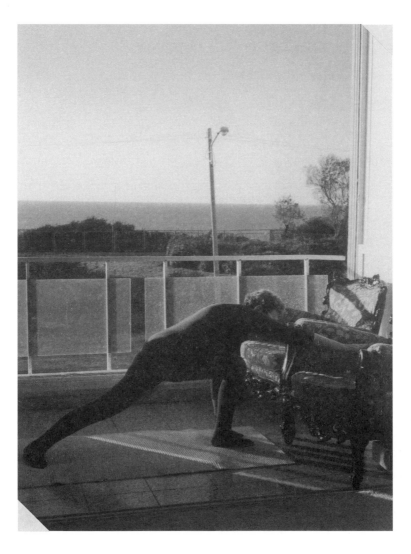

Repeat this exercise on the left:

- Stand with your legs wide apart (step position to the left). Inhale.
- Stretch your left arm out to the left.
- Turn your right arm backward (exhale).
- Remain in the stretch position for the count of 10.
- Place your left hand on the floor next to the outside of the left foot.
- Hold out your right foot forward in the direction of the left leg (inhale).
- Remain in this position for the count of 10 (exhale).
- Place your right hand on the back of your neck.
- Lift your left arm and stretch to the left (inhale).
- Bend your left knee.
- Your left elbow touches your right knee (exhale).

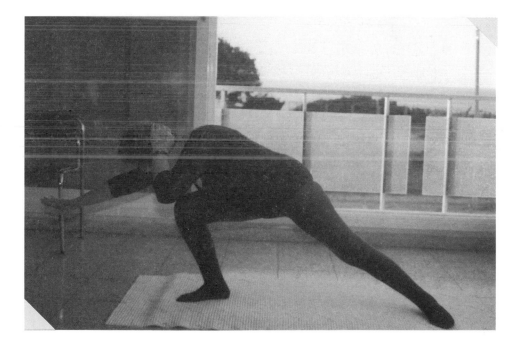

- Remain in this position for the count of 10.

- Straighten up (inhale).

- Move your left hand to your right ankle by turning your hip.

- Move your bent right arm behind your back (exhale).

- The back of your hand rests on your left hip.

- Remain in this position for the count of 10.

- Straighten up.

Repeat this movement twice on the left.

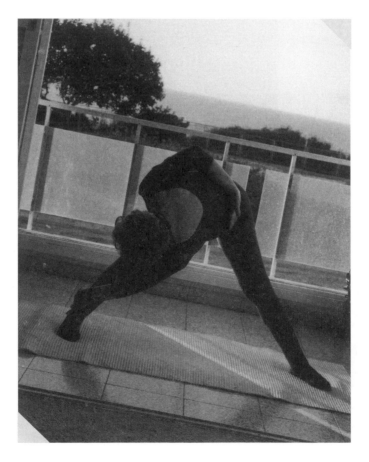

Treating the back of the body

- Stand up straight, legs together.
- Interlace your fingers behind your back in the region of your buttocks (inhale).
- Bend the upper part of your body forward.
- Lift your hands toward the ceiling (exhale). Inhale.
- Slide your interlaced hands along the back part of your legs until they reach your ankles.
  Your nose touches your knees.
  Your hands remain interlaced throughout the exercise.
- Release your hands (exhale).
- Straighten up vertebra by vertebra.
- Inhale.
- Bring your shoulder-blades close togcthcr and relax.
- Exhale.

Squeeze your shoulder-blades together three times.

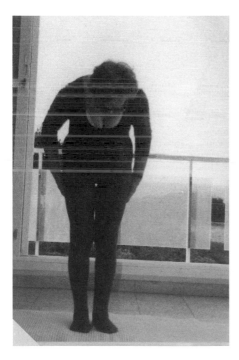
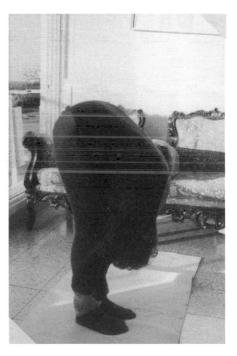

Bending forward (This exercise is for the spine)

- Stand up straight and erect, feet together.
- Lift your arms up straight and taut via the front of your body (inhale).
- Bend the upper part of your body forward, bending from the waist.

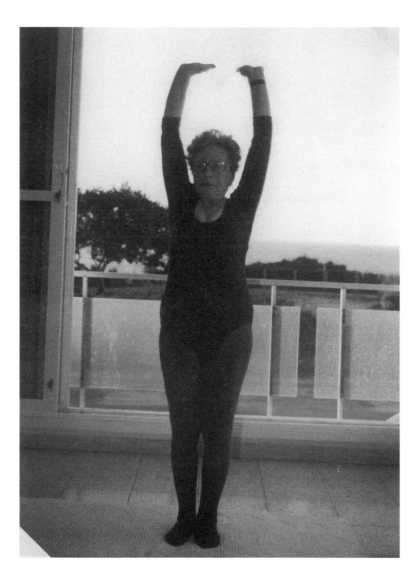

- Hold your ankles from the outside:
  Your thumb faces forward and your fingers face backward.
  Your nose touches your knees.
- Your arms are bent and gently pull the upper part of your body downward until your chest touches your thighs (exhale).
- Relax your body, and straighten up vertebra by vertebra. Inhale through your nose (exhale).

Do this exercise three times.

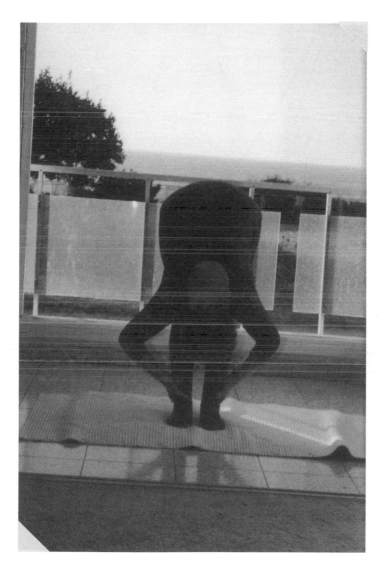

Sitting on a mattress

Positions for opening exercises

There are several starting positions for performing yoga exercises on a mattress:

– Sitting with your legs stretched forward, feet together.

– Sitting with your legs bent, feet on the mattress.

– Sitting cross-legged, knees bent and calves crossed in front of the body.

– Sitting sideways - right leg straight, left leg resting bent on the mattress, the sole of the left foot touching the inner right thigh, legs spread apart.

– Sitting with legs apart (a meter between the feet).

Lying on the mattress

– Lying on your back with your legs together, your arms straight down next to your body.

– Lying with your knees bent (soles of the feet on the mattress).

Other positions on the mattress

– Standing on all fours - number 1
Stand on your hands and knees, elbows taut and calves and feet on the mattress.

– Standing on all fours - number 2
Stand on your knees and forearms, elbows on the floor and calves and feet on the mattress.

- Kneeling
  Kneel. Your knees are bent and your calves are behind you on the mattress.
  The rest of your body is erect from the knees upward.

- Standing on your shoulders
  Lift your legs from the lying position toward the ceiling, and lift your
  back up off the floor. Your body is supported by your shoulders.

- Lying on your back
  Your legs are lifted from the pelvis.

Exercises lying on a mattress

Breathing: Inhale and exhale through your nose

Treating the tailbone

- Sit with your knees bent (inhale).
- Hold your knees:

  Your right hand holds your right knee, and your left hand holds your left knee.
- Rock from side to side.
- Lie down slowly: Start with the vertebrae closest to the buttocks, and slowly continue with the other vertebrae, one by one, while shifting your weight from side to side (exhale).
- Lie on your back with your knees bent, your feet on the floor.
- Take a deep abdominal breath.

  A kind of hollow is created in the lower back.
- Exhale while keeping the back on the floor.

Take three deep breaths.

Lengthening the spine

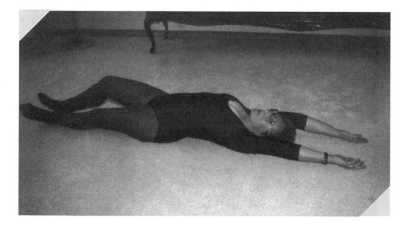

- Lie flat on your back (inhale).
- Lift your arms forward and upward.
- Stretch them above your head.
- Bend your knees. Your feet are on the floor.
- Bring your arms close to the knees, stretching forward.
- Your head rises while your chin is close to your chest.
  Your arms are between your legs (exhale).
- Straighten your legs, which are apart, and lift your feet to the ceiling.
  Your hands are stretched forward between your legs.

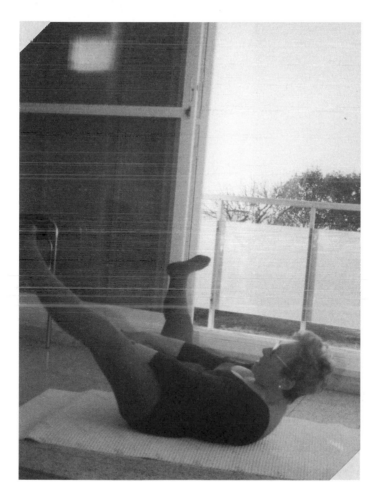

- Stretch your arms above your head (inhale). Bend your legs and place your feet on the floor.

- Lift your legs toward the ceiling, stretching them.
  You can lift your head.

- Hold your feet in your hands.
  Your legs are in the air.

- Your arms and legs are stretched upward (exhale).

- Straighten your legs, and lie flat on your back.

- Remain in this position for the count of five.

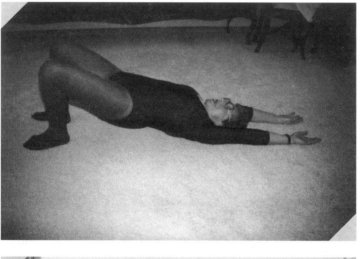

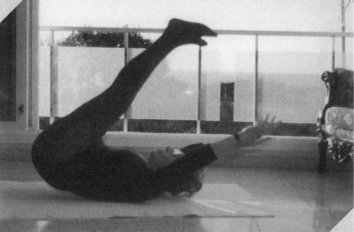

Exercise for making the body pliant

- Lie on your back.

- Interlace your fingers below the back of your neck (inhale).
  Your knees are bent, and your feet are on the floor.

- Contract your body by bending forward.

- Lift your head and bring your elbows and your knees close to one another
  (creating a kind of bird's nest).

- Try to touch your knees with your elbows (exhale).

- Straighten up.

Do this exercise three times.

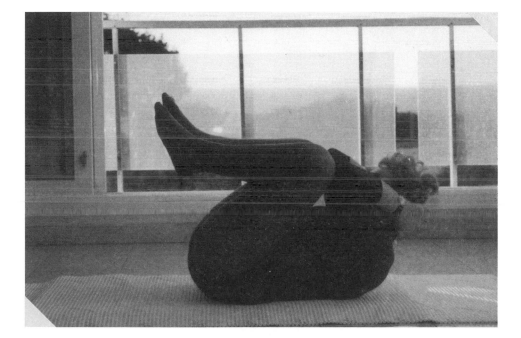

Releasing the lower back (continuation)

- Lie on your back (inhale), your arms stretched out above your head.

- Bend your knees.
  Your feet are on the floor.

- Gradually lift your buttocks as high as possible, vertebra by vertebra.

- Support yourself on your shoulders and on your feet.

- Remain in this position for the count of 30.

- Stretch your arms above your head.

- Slowly release your back, vertebra by vertebra (exhale).

Do this exercise three times.

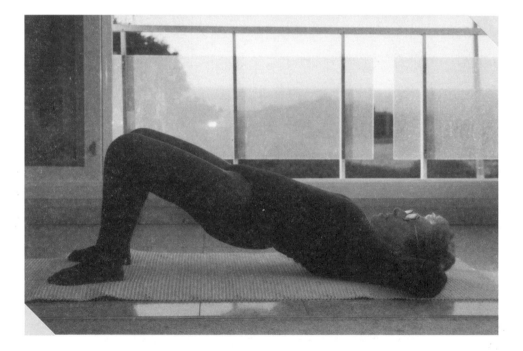

Strengthening the abdomen and making the back pliant

Knee to nose exercise

- Lie on your back (inhale).

- Lift your legs straight up.
  Your right hand grasps the back of your right knee, and your left hand grasps the back of your left knee.

- Lift your head slightly, and alternate bringing your left and right legs close to your nose.
  You can support the back of your knees with your hands (exhale).

Do 10 bends with each leg, alternately.

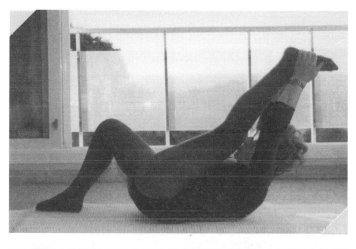

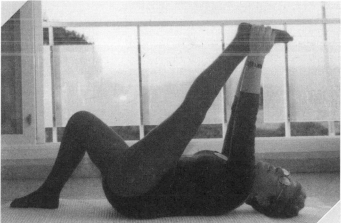

Bending forward
Exercise to conclude the set of exercises performed lying down

- Lie on your back with your legs together (inhale), your arms at your sides.
- Gently lift the upper part of your body.
- Grasp your feet, and straighten your legs by stretching forward. Your elbows are bent (exhale).

Do three stretches.

- Sit up (inhale).
- Bend forward again, further each time (exhale).

Do three bends.

- Place your hands on the lower part of your feet, on the outer side, and stretch your body forward.

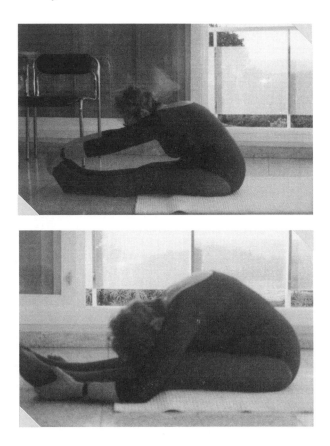

Exercises sitting on a mattress

Kidney twist - Stage 1

- Sit on the mattress in a one-sided position, your legs wide apart on the mattress, right leg straight at a 45-degree angle to your body, left leg bent at the knee, the sole of your left foot touching your right knee.
- Place your right hand on the back of your neck (inhale).
- Bend diagonally to the side, and stretch your right arm beyond your left knee (the right side of your body is stretched).
- Bring your right elbow close to your bent left knee (exhale). The upper part of your body twists to the left.
- Remain in this position for the count of 10 (inhale).
- Place your left arm, which is taut, on the outer side of your outstretched right leg. Stretch your left arm.
- Place your nose on your right knee and your chest on your right thigh.
- Exhale.
- Remain in this position for the count of 10.

Do this exercise five times.

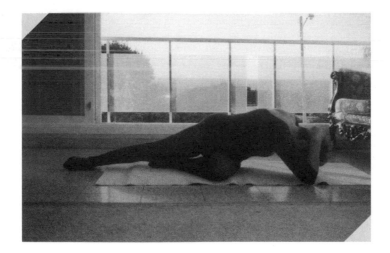

Repeat the exercise on the other side:

- Sit on the mattress in a one-sided position, your legs wide apart on the mattress, left leg straight at a 45-degree angle to your body, right leg bent at the knee, the sole of your right foot touching your left knee.

- Place your left hand on the back of your neck (inhale).

- Bend diagonally to the side, and stretch your left arm beyond your right knee (the left side of your body is stretched).

- Bring your left elbow close to your bent right knee (exhale).
  The upper part of your body twists to the right.

- Remain in this position for the count of 10 (inhale).

- Place your right arm, which is taut, on the outer side of your outstretched left leg. Stretch your right arm.

- Place your nose on your left knee and your chest on your left thigh.

- Exhale.

- Remain in this position for the count of 10.

Do this exercise five times.

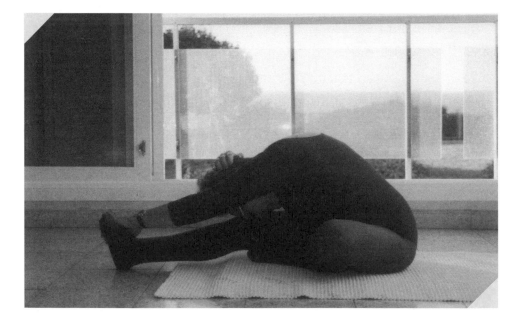

Exercise for effective kidney function - Stage 2

- Sit in the same one-sided position, your right leg straight and outstretched (inhale).

- Place your taut right arm in such a way that your fingers enclose the sole of your right foot from the inner side of the foot, and hold your foot as follows:

- Your arm is outstretched: Your thumb holds the top of your foot and the rest of your fingers hold the sole of your foot (you can hold it in the area of the pad next to the toes). If you find it difficult to get to, you can hold your right calf.

- Stretch your left arm from the side toward the right leg.

- Grasp your right foot from the outer side (your arms are crossed).

- Remain in this position for the count of 10 (exhale).

- Sit up.

Repeat this exercise on the other side:

- Sit in the same one-sided position, your left leg straight and outstretched (inhale). Place your taut left arm in such a way that your fingers enclose the sole of your left foot from the inner side of the foot, and hold your foot as follows:

- Your arm is outstretched: Your thumb holds the top of your foot and your fingers hold the sole of your foot (you can hold it in the area of the pad next to the toes). If you find it difficult to get to, you can hold your left calf.

- Stretch your right arm from the side toward the left leg.

- Grasp your left foot from the outer side (your arms are crossed).

- Remain in this position for the count of 10 (exhale).

- Sit up.

Getting the blood to flow in your legs

This can also be performed in a chair (as in the photo)

- Sit with your legs outstretched.
- Lift your right leg slightly above the floor.
- Place your right hand below your right knee.
- Place your left hand below the calf muscle of your right leg.
- Stick your heel out.
- Your toes move toward your calf.
- Remain in this position for 10 seconds.
- Straighten your right foot ballerina style.
- Remain in this position for the count of 10.

Do this exercise three times.

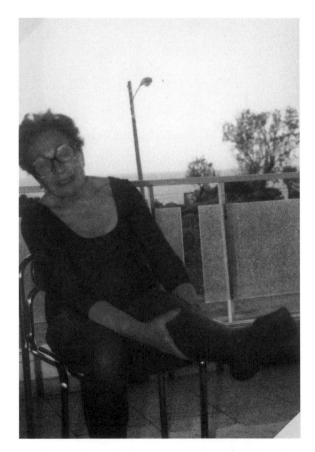

Repeat the exercise on the other side:

- Sit with your legs outstretched.
- Lift your left leg slightly above the floor.
- Place your left hand below your left knee.
- Place your right hand below the calf muscle of your left leg.
- Stick your heel out.
- Your toes move toward your calf.
- Remain in this position for 10 seconds.
- Straighten your left foot ballerina style.
- Remain in this position for the count of 10.

Do this exercise three times.

This exercise helps the flow of blood in the leg. You can feel how the muscle draws the blood from the foot.

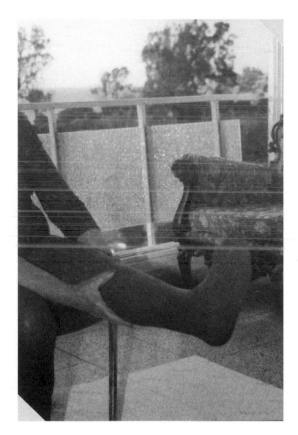

Treating the upper part of the spine by lifting the head

- Sit with your legs outstretched.
- Place your hands behind your head, above the nape. Your hands support your head (inhale).
- Lift your head slightly, and let it go gently (exhale).

Do this movement three times.

- Place your hands behind your head (inhale).
  Your fingers point toward your neck, and your elbows face the ceiling.
- Move your chin toward your chest (exhale), and lift your head.

Do this movement three times.

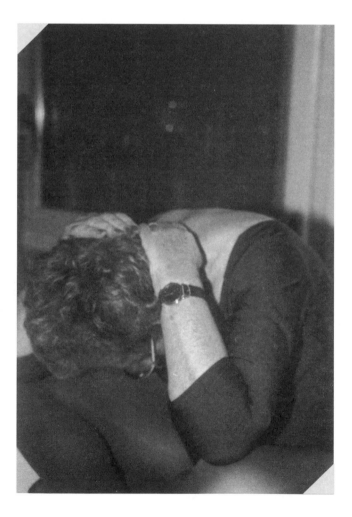

Bending forward for pliancy
Exercise to conclude the sitting exercises

- Sit with your legs outstretched.

- Take a deep abdominal breath through your nose, and stretch your body. Lift your arms straight above your head.

- Bend forward and hold your outer ankles in your hands, your thumbs pointing forward, and your fingers behind the ankles.

- Bring your nose as close as possible to your knees, with your chest on your thighs (exhale).

Do this exercise three times.

Between exercises, relax your body.

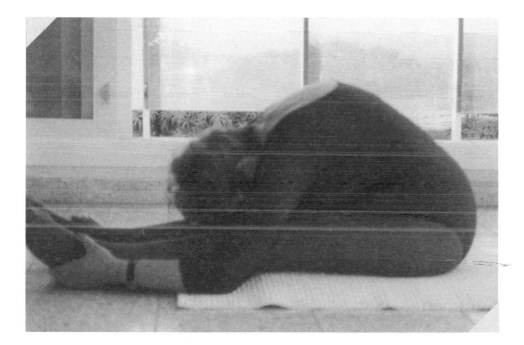

Self-massage

Massage for the spine

- Lie on your back on the mattress.

- Bend your knees on your body.

- Place your hands behind your thighs, and roll forward and backward five times, alternately, in the direction of the feet and in the direction of the head. (Your feet serve as a lever that pulls you forward to a sitting position.)

- Lie on your back (inhale).

- Stretch your arms upward, and stretch your legs, too, while pushing your heels downward (exhale).

- Place your hands at the sides of your body, relaxed and resting.

Recommendation for relaxation

> Relaxation completes the activity in the yoga method.

Our lives are full of tension. Tension and nervousness cause a great deal of damage to the body.

Tension is our enemy.

Free yourself of tension!

Don't spend your life suffering from troubles that cannot be cured!

Drain them from your body!

Live the moment, and exploit it for your benefit!

> Relaxing for 10 minutes is the equivalent of two hours' sleep.

Contraction and relaxation for deep relaxation

- Lie on your back.

- Contract your organs in sequence, from your tailbone to your head, and then relax them in turn.

- You can feel every vertebra resting on the floor, your spine long, pliant, and relaxed.

- Your body becomes heavy and relaxed, and does not permit you to move.

- Your chest is relaxed, your face and your tongue are relaxed.

- Your eyes are relaxed.

- Your brain is relaxed - devoid of thoughts.

- Your breath says: Relax... relax...

- Your abdomen is relaxed.

- Your arms are heavy, your legs are heavy.

- Your ears are impervious to sounds from the outside.

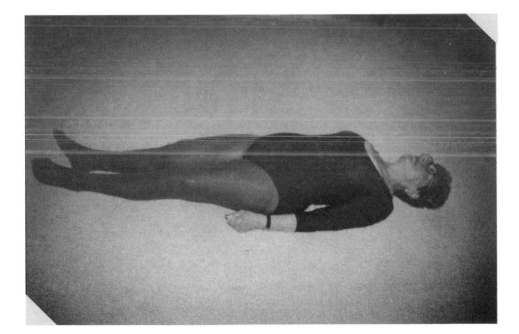

- The relaxation is total.
- Your breathing is relaxed and calm.

Continue like this for about 12 minutes.

When you have completed the relaxation, rouse your body very slowly:

- Gently wiggle your toes and fingers.
  Curl up like a fetus on your left side.
  Roll over, via your back, to your right side and curl up.
  Remain on each side for a few minutes.
  Decide for yourself how long to remain in this position.

- Wake up relaxed, and open your eyes for a second or two. You let the light and colors penetrate you.

- Close your eyes, and then open them again.

- Each time, let more and more colors penetrate your body (using visualization).

- Try to look on the bright side of life.
  "Don't cry over spilt milk - the cat will lick it up."
  May we all have a day full of happiness and good energy.

- Slowly get up into a sitting position and continue to rise, back curved, vertebra by vertebra, until you are standing.

In the yoga method, every part of your body works;

even the roots of your hair are treated.

Self-massage for the back

- Clench your fist.
  Your thumb joint serves as an instrument of pressure.

- Place your right thumb joint into the hollow of the left side of your clavicle, next to your neck.
  Your left hand supports the arm that is exerting pressure - it holds the elbow of the arm that is exerting pressure.

- Press the painful points while exhaling until you feel the pain subsiding.

- Place your left thumb joint into the hollow of the right side of your clavicle, next to your neck.

- Your right hand supports the arm that is exerting pressure - it holds the.

- Press the painful points while exhaling until you feel the pain subsiding.

- Massage the back of your neck behind your ears and relax.

- The blood flows to your head better.

> **We help our body heal itself when we convince**
>
> **ourselves of the following:**
>
> **From moment to moment, from hour to hour,**
>
> **from day to day, I feel better and better in every way.**

Strengthening the knees and the back

- Stand on all fours - position number 2.

- Stand on your knees, the top of your feet and your elbows (inhale).

- Lift your feet off the floor.
  Your knees serve as a lever.

- Put your feet on the floor again.

- Straighten your arms and stretch them. Your hands are on the floor.

- Stretch your entire body from your hands to your tailbone.

- Remain in this position for the count of 10 (exhale).

- Go back to standing on all fours.

Do this exercise three times.

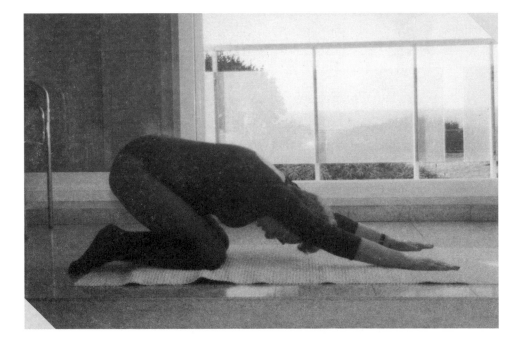

Making the spine pliant - the cat exercise

Stage 1

- Stand on all fours - position number 1.
  Your hands, knees, and top of your feet are on the mattress.

- Lift your head and inhale.

- Press your abdomen downward, and let your back sink.

- Put your chin on your chest, and exhale.

- Curve your back and contract your abdominal muscles.

- Breathe deeply, and raise your buttocks. In effect, you are standing on your hands and feet. Your buttocks are in the air (creating a kind of tent).

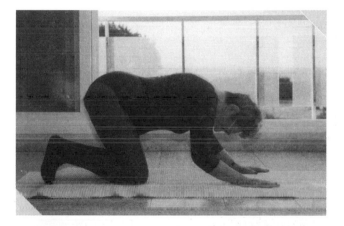

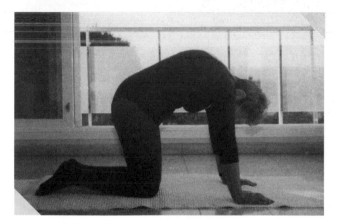

- In the stretch from your feet to your hands, you do not change your location.
  Both your arms and your legs are straight and taut.

- Try to touch the floor with your heels.
  Your entire body is stretched - particularly the tendons of your legs.
  You can feel your spine (exhale).

- Relax your body.

- In this position (like a cat), stretch and relax your two legs alternately with a light backward stretch: gently straighten and bend your knees.

Do this stretch about 10 times, alternately and quickly.

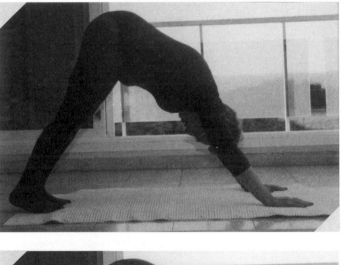

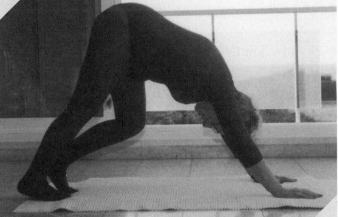

Stage 2 - Diagonal stretch for balance

- Stand on all fours - position number 1, and relax your body. Inhale through your nose.
- Stretch your right arm forward in the air, and stretch your left leg backward. Stretch your fingers and toes (exhale).
- Resume the all-fours position.
  Do this exercise 10 times with your left arm and your right leg.
- Relax.

Stage 3 - Stretching and making the spine pliant

- Stand on all fours - position number 1 (inhale).
- Stretch your arms forward.
  Place your hands on the floor.
- Place your forearms on the floor.
- Bend forward on your forearms and on your knees.
- Lift your feet off the floor (exhale).
- Remain in this position for the count of five.
- Place your feet on the floor (inhale).
  Your hands do not move.
- Stretch your buttocks backward (exhale).
  Do this exercise five times.

Stage 4 - Bending backward and making the spine pliant

- Kneel (inhale).
- Lift your arms and stretch them upward. The palms of your hands face each other.
- From the shoulder joint, turn each arm once upward and backward in a big circle.
- Grasp your heels from behind.
- This results in an arched back (exhale).
- Sit on your ankles.
- Relax.
- Place your hands on the floor at the sides of your body, the back of your hands next to your feet. Bend down and place your forehead on the floor.
- Relax.

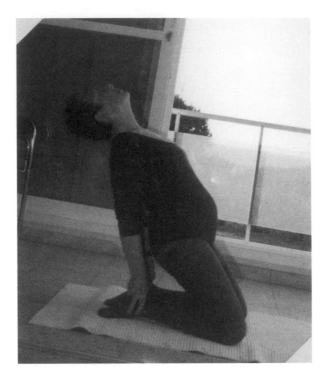

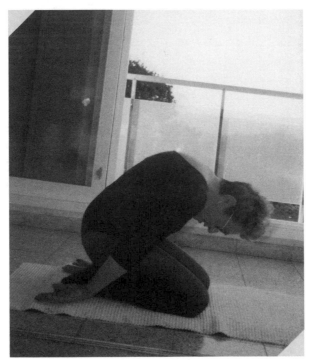

Repeat the exercise:

- Kneel once again, stretch, stretch your arms upward, turn your arms upward and backward once.

- Stretch your arms behind your legs, with your hands on the floor and the fingers facing backward.

- Sit on your ankles, and relax.

- Place your hands behind you, along your legs.

- Bend over, and place your forehead on the floor.
  You can feel your spine resting. Relax.

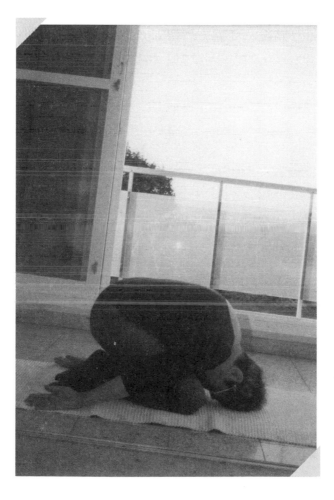

Stage 5 - Treating the lower back

- Stand on all fours - position number 1, and breathe deeply. Relax the tension.
- Lift your right knee in the direction of your nose, and straighten your bent leg backward.
- Lift your ankle in the direction of the ceiling.
- Let your bent leg move through the air to the right, and bring it back to its place.

Do this exercise five times.

Repeat the exercise with the left leg:
- Lift your left knee in the direction of your nose, and straighten your bent leg backward.
- Lift your ankle in the direction of the ceiling.
- Let your bent leg move through the air to the left, and bring it back to its place.

Do this exercise five times.

Stage 6 - Turning the thigh joints

- Stand on all fours - position number 1 (inhale).
- Bring your right knee close to your right elbow.
- Move your right knee in a turn to the right, backward, and forward, and bring it back in a circle in the direction of the elbow (exhale).

Do this exercise five times.

- Inhale, bend your toes, and bend your knee.
- Lift your right leg toward your nose.
- Lift it, bent, backward, with the heel facing upward.

Do this five times at a fast pace, and relax. (Exhale.)

Repeat the exercise with the other foot (inhale).
- Bring your left knee close to your left elbow.
- Move your left knee in a turn to the left, backward, and forward, and bring it back in a circle in the direction of the elbow (exhale).

Do this exercise five times.

- Bend your toes, and bend your knee (inhale).

- Lift your left leg toward your nose.

- Lift it, bent, backward, with the heel facing upward (exhale).

Do this five times at a fast pace, and relax.

Stage 7 - From standing on all fours to standing erect

- Stand on all fours - position number 1.

- Bend your toes upward so that they face the knees (inhale).

- Lift yourself up to a tent position: Your hands and feet are on the floor, and your buttocks are raised. Your arms and legs are straight and taut.

- Stretch your heels toward the floor.

- Stretch and relax both legs simultaneously. Stretch and relax 10 times.

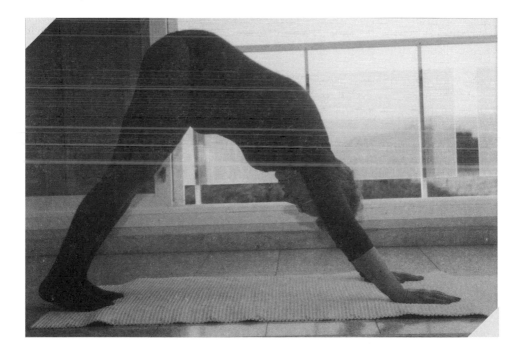

- Move your feet in tiny steps toward your hands, until your feet and hands meet (inhale).
- Place your chin on your chest and contract your abdominal muscles.
- Lift your knees, contract your lower front thigh muscles upward.

  The muscle is stretched from the knee upward. Relax. (The thigh muscles lift your knees.)
- Contract and relax 10 times for the count of 10 each time.
- Release the abdominal muscles (exhale).
- Gradually straighten up, vertebra by vertebra, from bottom to top.
- Lift your arms and stretch your entire body upward.

Stage 8 - Bending forward

- Stand up straight with your legs together (inhale).
- Stretch your arms forward and upward, with the palms of your hands forward, bend forward from the waist, and grasp your ankles (or higher). Your thumbs are in front, your fingers are behind, and your legs are straight.
- Pull your elbows while bending them to the side.
- The pull stretches the body downward (exhale).
- Straighten up carefully, vertebra by vertebra, and relax.

Do this exercise three times.

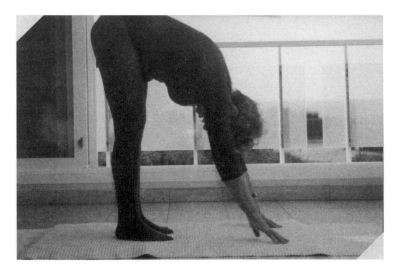

Exercises lying on a mattress

Leg exercises with body stretching

- Sit on the mattress.
- Lie down gradually, vertebra by vertebra, until your back is on the floor (inhale).
- Lift your hands above your head.
- Point your feet like a ballerina and stretch, then relax (exhale).
- Inhale and push your elbows, stretching your arms. Relax (exhale).

Repeat the exercise, alternately, five times.

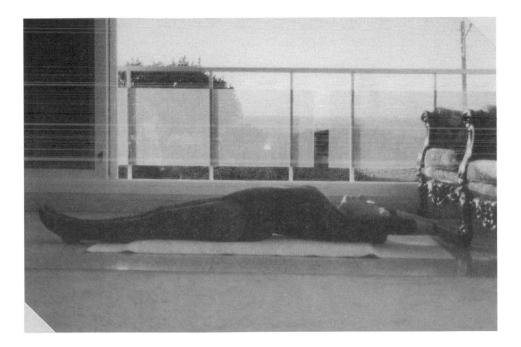

Contracting and relaxing

- Lie on your back, your arms at your sides.

- Inhale deeply through your nose.

- Contract your entire body.

- Remain in that position for the count of 10, and relax.

- You mainly contract your back and your buttocks, and then relax.

- Exhale.

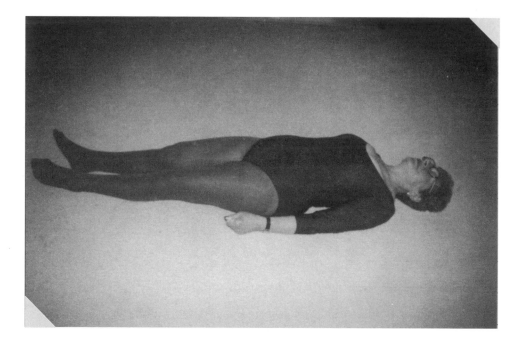

The shoulder stand - the princess of yoga

This exercise can be performed in two ways:

a. For people who suffer from high blood pressure and menstruating women:
   - Lie on your entire back (inhale).
   - Lift your legs to a 90-degree angle, your feet facing the ceiling.

b. Other people:
   - Lie on your back (inhale).
   - Lift up your entire back up to the nape.
     Your arms remain in their place on the mattress.
     You can use your hands to support your back.

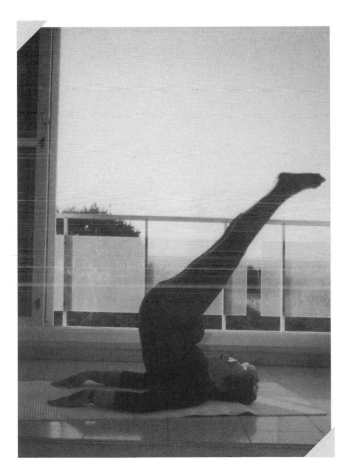

In the various positions (on the back or on the shoulders), you do the following exercises:

- Take relaxed breaths throughout the exercises.
- Move your feet up and down. Straighten your legs simultaneously. Your toes point toward your face, in the direction of the body.
- Point your feet like a ballerina, and push your heels so that your toes approach your body.

Repeat the movement 10 times, quickly.

- Turn both feet around at the ankles.

Turn them to the right 10 times and to the left 10 times.

Repeat the previous movement:

- Move your feet.
- Point your feet like a ballerina, and push your heels so that your toes approach your body.
- The movement is performed quickly and alternately (exhale).

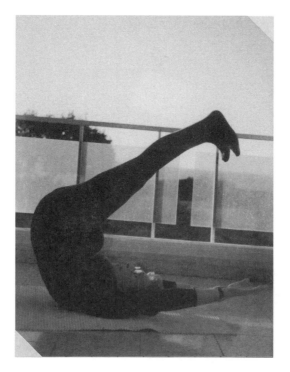

Leg stretching

Position 1: Shoulder stand

- Place your taut right leg on the floor above your head.
  Your left leg remains straight up.
- Switch leg positions:
  Your right leg goes up, and your left leg goes down toward the floor above your head, simultaneously.

Do this exercise three times on each side.

- During the exercise, take relaxed breaths, and at the end of the exercise, both legs point straight up toward the ceiling.
- Bend your right leg slightly toward your nose.
  Your left leg remains stretched up in the air.
- Switch leg positions:
  Your right leg goes up, and your left leg goes down toward your nose, simultaneously.

Do this exercise 10 times.

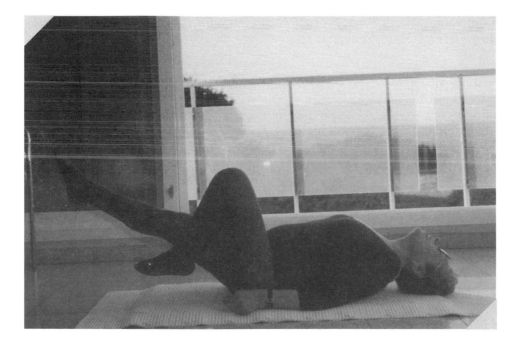

Position 2: On the entire back

- Place your straight, taut right leg on the floor.
  Your left leg remains straight up at a 90-degree angle to the body.
- Switch leg positions:
  Your right leg goes up, and your left leg goes down toward the floor, simultaneously.

Do this exercise three times on each side.

- Bend your right leg slightly toward your nose.
  Your left leg remains stretched up in the air.
- Switch leg positions:
  Your right leg goes up, and your left leg goes down toward your nose, simultaneously.
- During the exercise, take relaxed breaths.
- At the end of the exercise, both legs point straight up toward the ceiling.

Do this exercise 10 times.

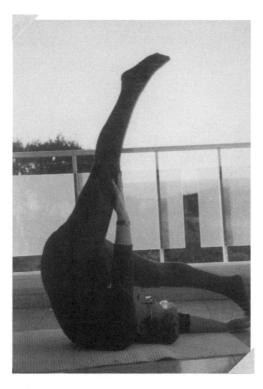

Stretching the entire body - plow

- Lie on your back (inhale).
- Lift your legs up toward the ceiling.
- Hold your feet by the toes.
- Remain in this position for the count of five (exhale).
- Move your legs slightly apart.

Your hands are still holding your feet.

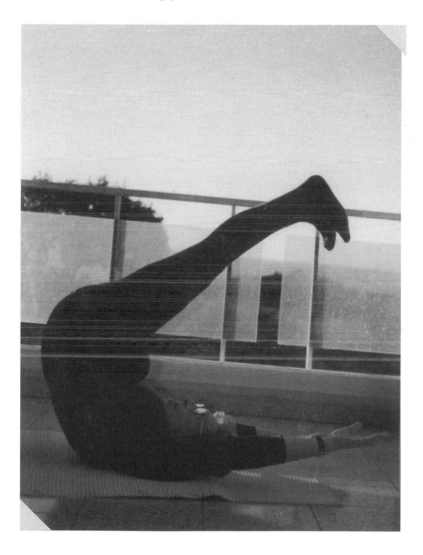

Position 1: Shoulder stand

- Inhale and bring both legs and the hands holding them over your head (exhale).

- Remain in this position for the count of 10 (exhale).

- Lower your back onto the mattress, vertebra by vertebra, one leg after the other.

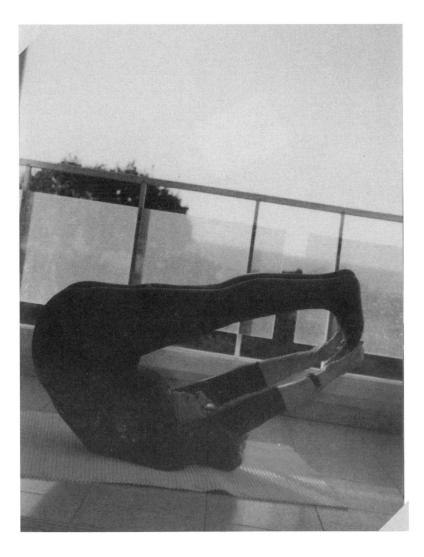

The exercise is also suitable for position 2, which begins by lying on your back:

- Slowly put your legs down when they are straight.

- Stretch your arms forward, having let go of your feet (in the opposite direction to your legs). Now you are in a "sitting" position. Stretch and relax the tension in your body.

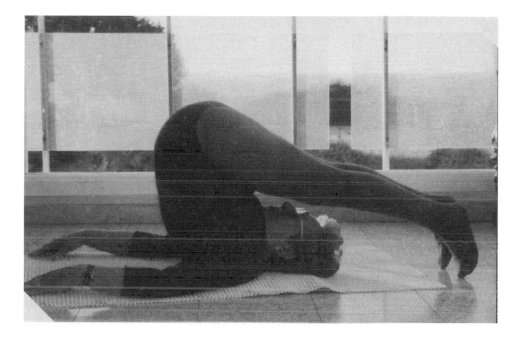

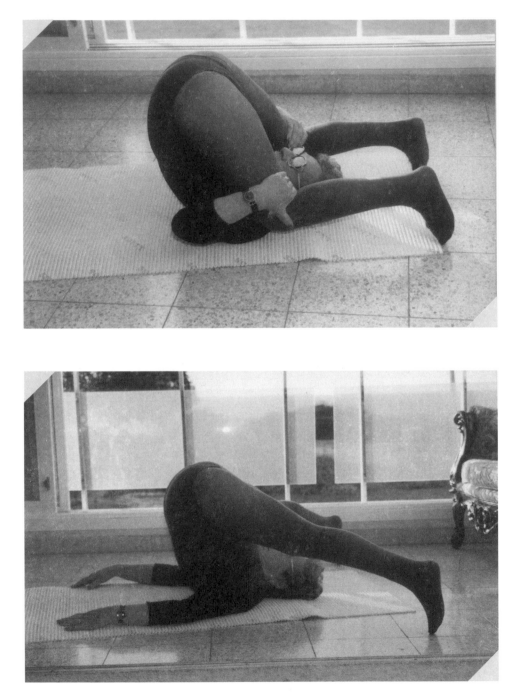

Bending forward

- Lie on your back (inhale).

- Stretch your arms forward, and pull your body to a sitting position.

- Lift your arms, and stretch them forward to grasp your ankles.
  Your thumb faces forward, and the rest of your fingers face backward.

- Bend your elbows and pull them sideways.
  This movement causes the body to stretch (exhale).

- Lift your arms again, inhaling. Once more, hold your ankles and stretch.

- Exhale.

Do three stretches.

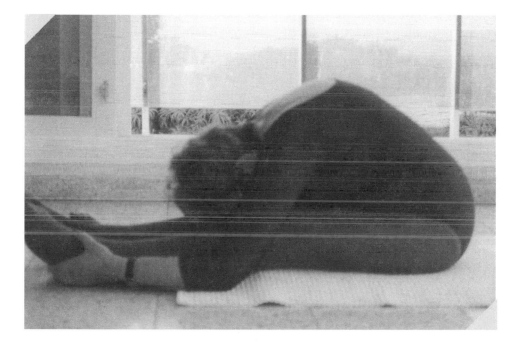

Exercises for the arms sitting down

Breathing: Inhale and exhale through your nose.

- Warm your hands like this:
  Place your forearms next to your ribs, with your palms relaxed and touching each other. Rub them together.
- Sit with outstretched legs or cross-legged (inhale).
- Bend over and stretch your arms forward.
  Your hands touch at the thumbs.
  Your palms face the floor.
- Stretch your right arm forward, then stretch your left arm forward, and so on (exhale).

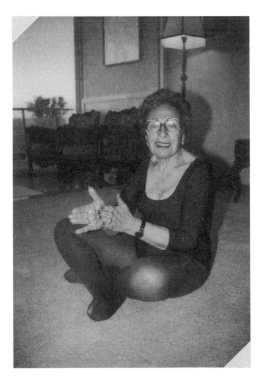

Arm stretching

- Sit with outstretched legs and interlace your fingers (exhale).
- Inhale.
- Stretch your arms forward, and turn your hands so that the inner side of your interlaced hands is away from your body.
- Push your hands forward and stretch.
- Remain in this position for the count of five (exhale).

Do the exercise three times.

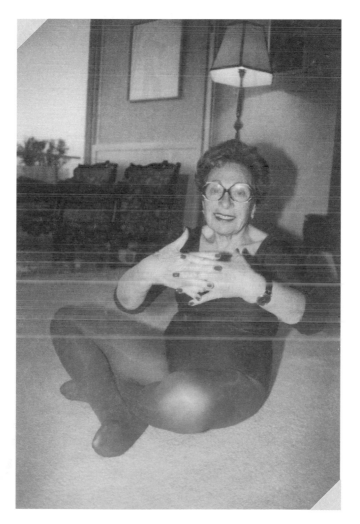

Contracting the shoulder-blades

- Interlace your fingers behind your back (inhale).
  Your palms face upward, and your arms are straight.

- Stretch your hands backward and downward, toward the floor.

- Bring your shoulder-blades close to each other.

- Remain in this position for the count of five, exhale and relax.

Do this movement twice.

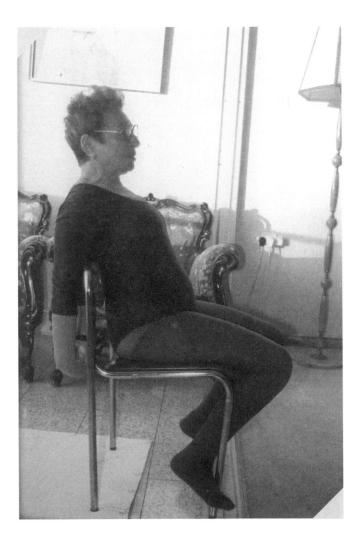

Arm twists

- Sit with outstretched legs.

- Cross your arms as follows:
  Your right arm over your left arm, your hands facing each other.

- Interlace your fingers (inhale).

- Stretch your arms.

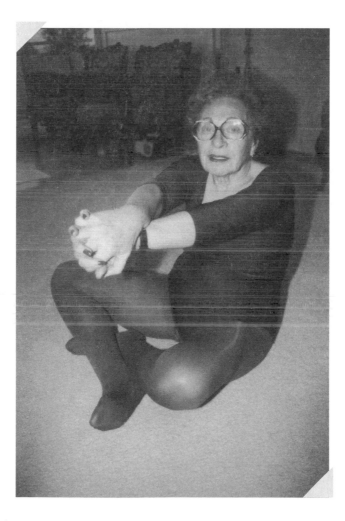

- Bend your elbows, bring your interlaced hands close to your chest, and lift them up toward your face.

- Exhale.

- Do not release your fingers.

- Bring your arms back to their initial position, that is, stretched forward with hands interlaced.

Do this exercise three times.

Repeat this exercise three times, crossing your left arm over your right arm.

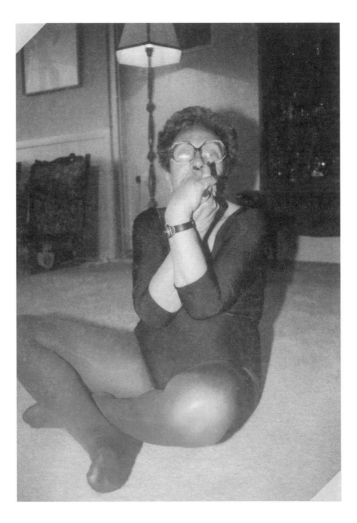

Stretching the arms

- Sit with outstretched legs.

- Stretch your arms forward.
  Your hands both face the floor.

- Place your right hand on your left hand, interlace your fingers, and bend your left hand inward. One hand presses the other (the palm of your right hand presses on the back of your left hand).

Do this movement five times.

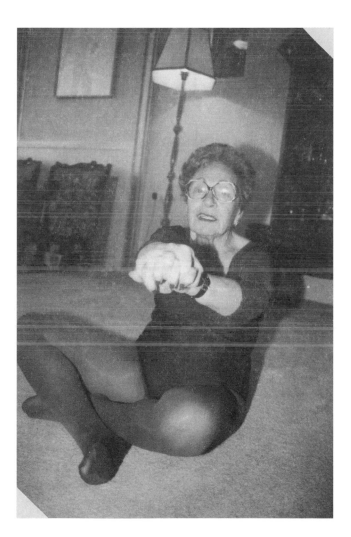

- Change the hand position as follows:
  Place your left hand on your right hand and interlace your fingers.

Do this movement five times.

- Rub your hands together as you did at the beginning of the arm exercises.

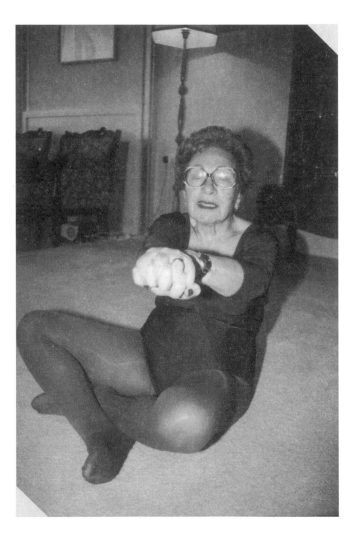

Quick release of tension

- Place your hands on your clavicle as follows:
  Your right hand is placed on the right side of the clavicle.
  Your left hand is placed on the left side of the clavicle.

- Inhale and throw your arms outward and downward.
  Your palms face upward.
  The movement resembles that of brushing dirt off the body.

- Put your hands back on your clavicle.

Do this movement quickly five times (exhale).

- Place your hands on your clavicle.
  Your hands do not leave the clavicle; turn both elbows abruptly once outward and once inward, like a butterfly movement.

Do this movement five times forward and five times backward.

Strengthening the hand

- Your hands touch each other, with their roots near to your sternum, and your fingers facing forward.

- Your hands press each other.

- Press your fingertips while moving the roots of your hands apart.

- Remain in this position for the count of five.

- Press the roots of your hands and your pinkies and thumbs open the rest of the fingers like the petals of a flower.

- Remain in this position for the count of five.

Do this exercise in the first way and in the second way, alternately, three times.

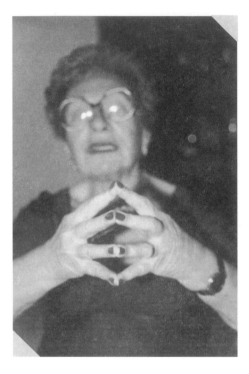

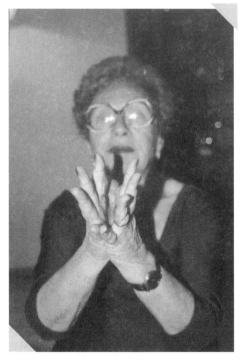

Exercises for the neck sitting down

Stage 1

- Sit with outstretched legs (inhale).
- Turn and look to the right (exhale).
- Inhale and turn and look to the left (exhale).

Do this exercise 10 times.

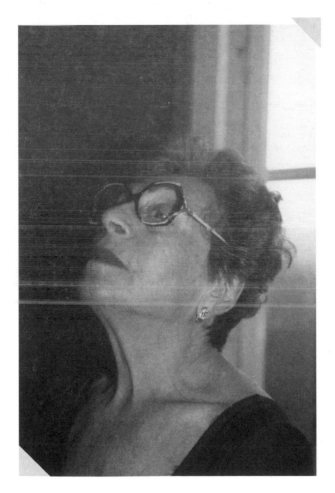

Stage 2

- Look ahead.

- Inhale, lift your head and look upward.

- Bring your chin close to your chest, look downward (exhale).

Do this exercise five times.

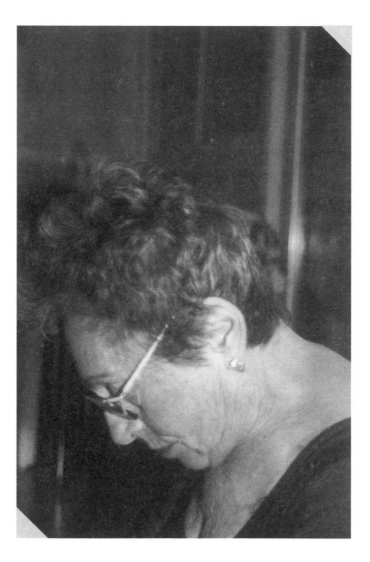

Stage 3

- Inhale and place your right ear on your right shoulder (exhale).
- Inhale and place your left ear on your left shoulder (exhale).

Do this exercise five times.

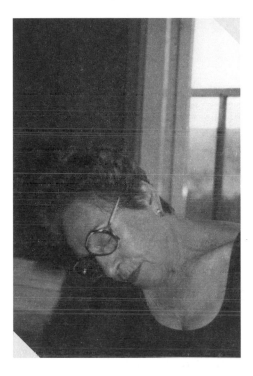

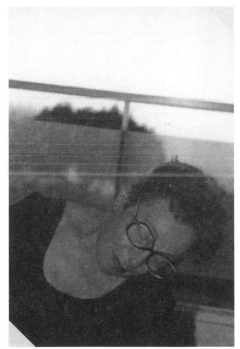

Stage 4

- Bring your chin close to your chest.

- Turn your head gently and slowly in big circles to the right, then upward, then to the left, then downward.

Do this exercise five times on each side.

- At the conclusion of these exercises, massage the back of your neck behind your ears in order to dispel the tension and to get the blood to flow to your head.

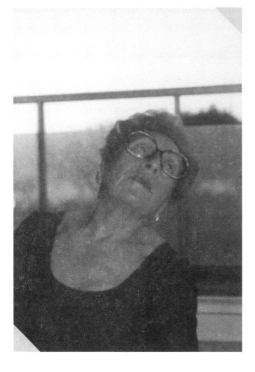

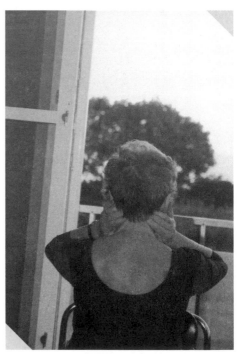

Breathing exercises

For cleaning out the air openings in the body

- Sit comfortably on a chair or on the floor.
- Blow your nose thoroughly.
- Use your right thumb to block your right nostril.
- Take a deep abdominal breath through your left nostril, with your mouth closed.
- Use two fingers to block your left nostril as well.
- Hold the air in your lungs for the count of eight.

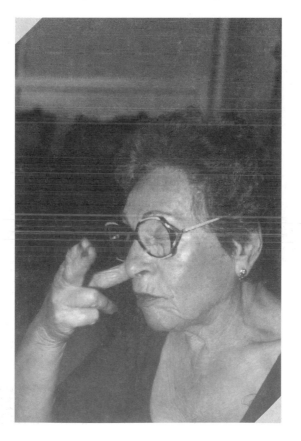

- Release your right nostril and exhale the air through it to the count of eight.

- Continue blocking your left nostril with your left thumb.

- Take a deep abdominal breath through your right nostril, with your mouth closed.

- Use two fingers to block your right nostril as well.

- Hold the air in your lungs for the count of eight.

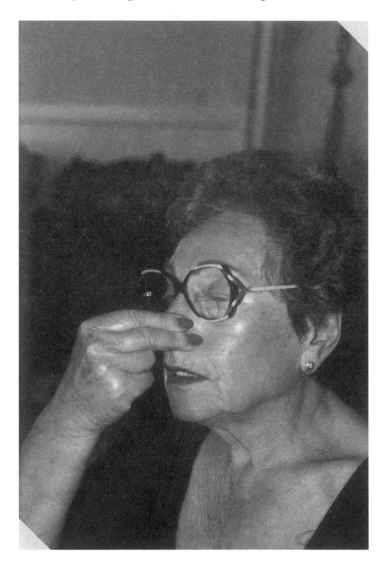

- Release your left nostril and exhale the air through it to the count of eight.

A kind of circle of breathing is created.

Do this exercise five times.

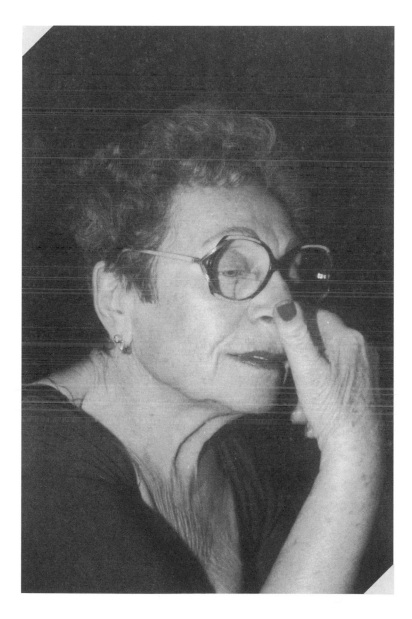

Chest breathing

- Place your hands on your chest.

- Your fingertips touch one another.

- Lift your elbows sideways at a 90-degree angle to your body.

- Breathe chest breathing - your ribs and shoulders rise up.

- Breathe to the count of eight.

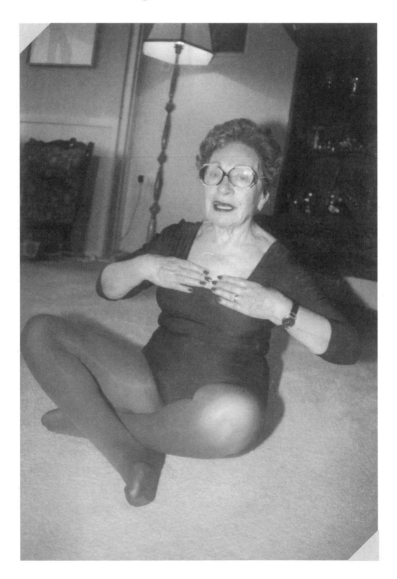

- Move your hands away from each other on your chest.

- Hold your breath for the count of eight.

- Release the air to the count of eight.

- Bring your hands together once again.

Do this exercise five times.

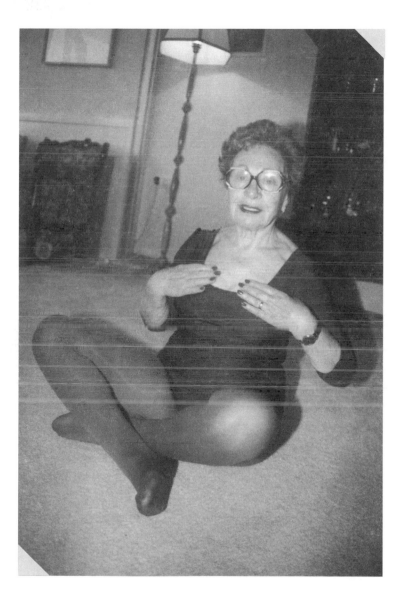

Abdominal breathing

- Place your hands on your abdomen, slightly below the diaphragm.

- Breathe through your nose to the count of eight, while lifting your elbows and filling your abdomen with air.

- Hold your breath for the count of eight.

- While lowering your elbows, exhale through your nose to the count of eight.

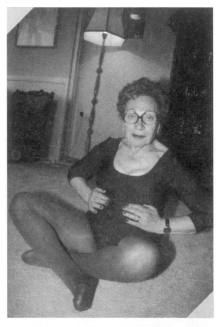

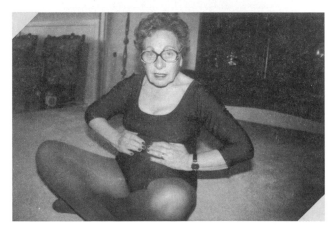

Exercises for the face

The principle of these exercises is to stretch and contract the facial muscles alternately in a particular area of the face. The exercises are performed sitting down.

Stage 1

- Chant the vowel "e" continuously while pulling your lower jaw forward and upward.

- Remain in this position for the count of eight.

Do this exercise three times.

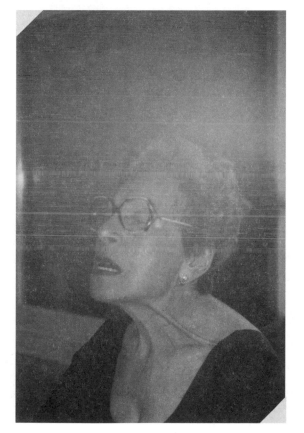

Stage 2

- Chant the vowel "o" continuously, with rounded lips.
- Remain in this position for the count of eight.

Do this exercise three times.

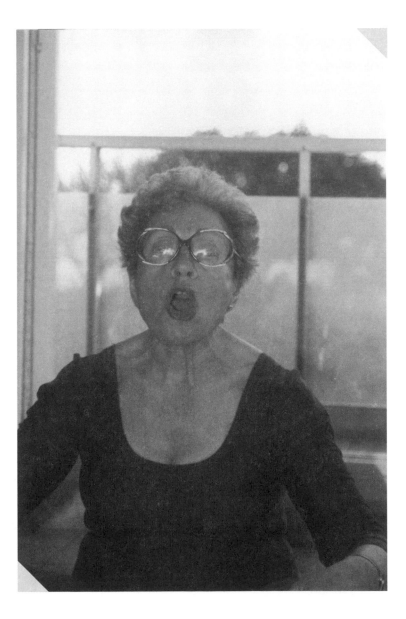

Stage 3

- Chant the vowel "u".
- Remain in this position for the count of eight.

Do this exercise three times.

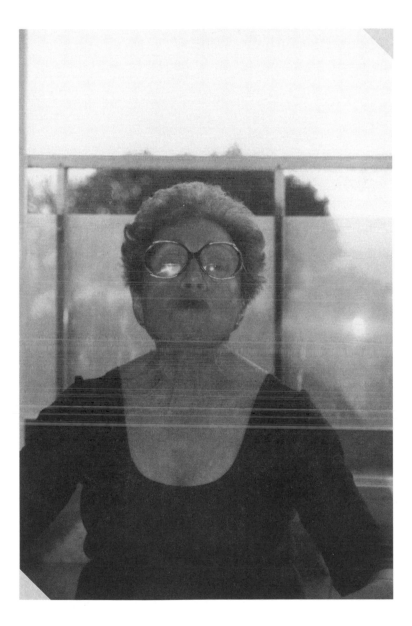

Stage 4

- Chant the vowel "i" by pulling your lips sideways.

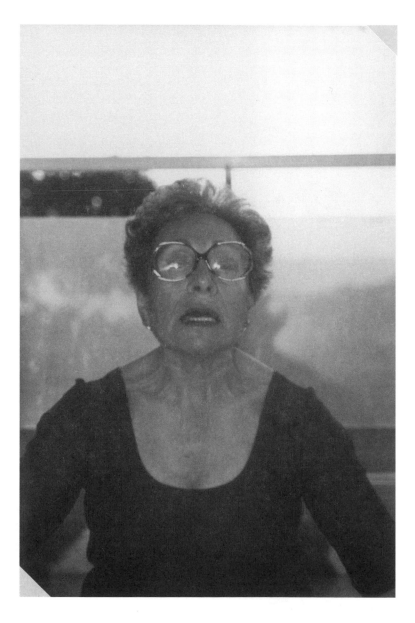

Stage 5

- While pulling your lower jaw upward and pulling your chest down, chant the syllable "oum".

  This stretches the neck.

  If you look in a mirror, you see your neck tendons protruding.

  You can also touch your neck and feel this.

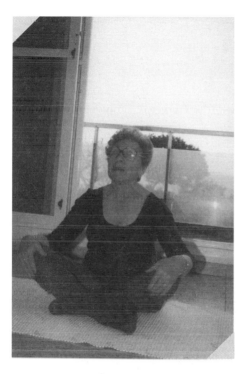

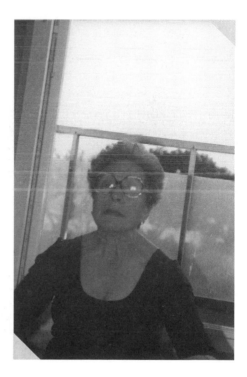

Treating the ears

These exercises are performed sitting down.

- Place your index fingers behind your ears.
- Move your ears without using your fingers.

You must do these exercises many times until these muscles are strengthened.

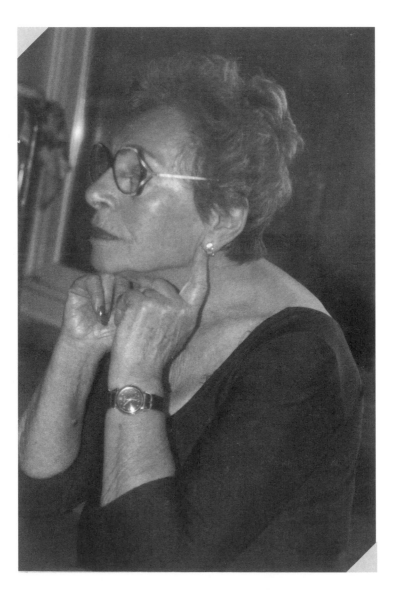

Strengthening the jaw muscles and releasing them

- The exercises are performed sitting down.
- Close your mouth and fill it with air.
- The right side of your face protrudes.
- Move the air to your left cheek.
- The fingers of your right hand help push the air to the left.
- The left cheek protrudes.
- Relax.

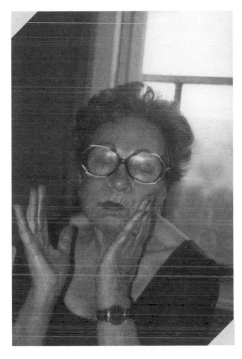 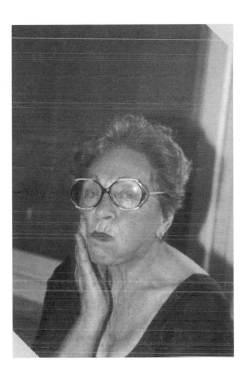

Massage of the face, mouth, and tongue

The exercise is performed sitting down.

- Roll your tongue around your mouth in a clockwise circular movement. The tip of the tongue presses on all the inner regions of the mouth.
- Switch directions.

Do this exercise five times, alternately.

Exercises for the eyes

The exercises help improve vision and prevent cataracts (blurred lens and a white spot on the cornea).

The exercises are performed sitting down, without moving your head.

- Roll your eyes up and down 10 times.

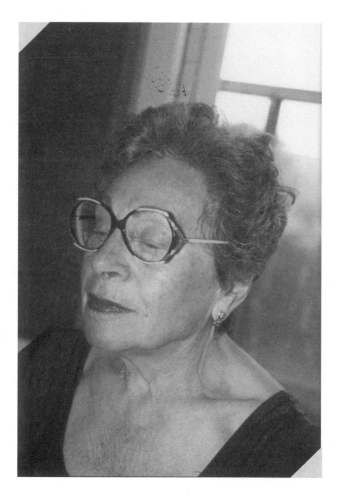

- Roll your eyes right and left 10 times.

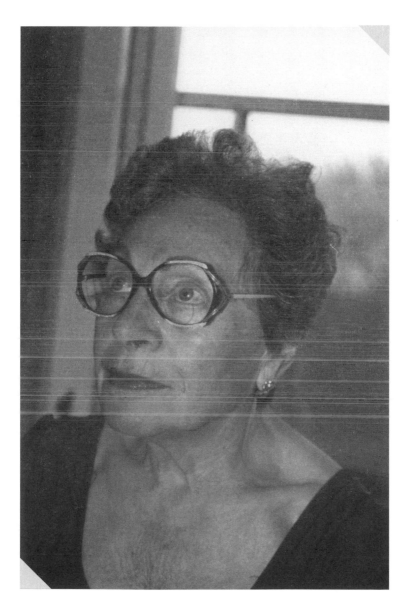

- Look diagonally 10 times:

  First to the right-hand corner of the ceiling, and then behind you to the left-hand corner of the floor.

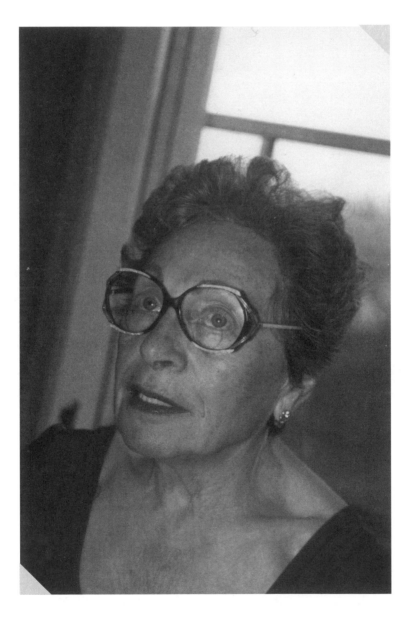

- Look diagonally 10 times:

  First to the left-hand corner of the ceiling, and then behind you to the right-hand corner of the floor.

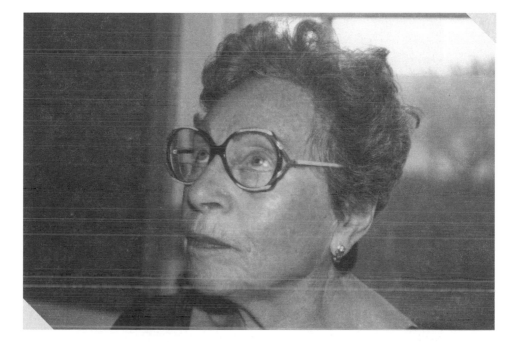

Eye exercise using the fingers

The exercise is performed sitting down.

- Hold your index finger at a distance of 20 cm from your eyes.

- Stare at it and try to see a double finger.

In order to succeed at the exercise, focus your vision on a distance of a meter or two beyond the finger.

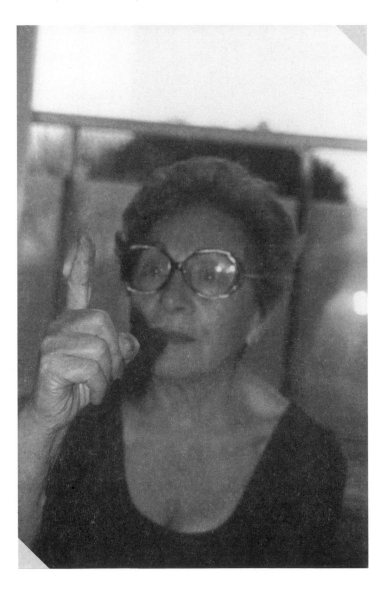

Eye exercise in conjunction with the third eye

The third eye is located in the center of the forehead above the nose.

- Look upward at your third eye.
  You can put your finger on your third eye.

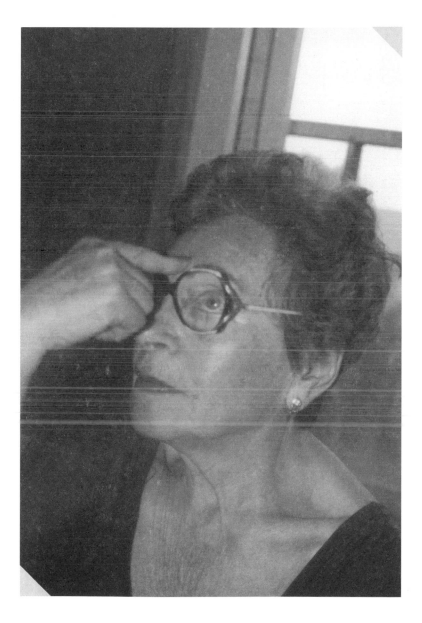

- Move your gaze down to the tip of your nose.

  This results in a kind of squint.

Do this exercise three times, alternately.

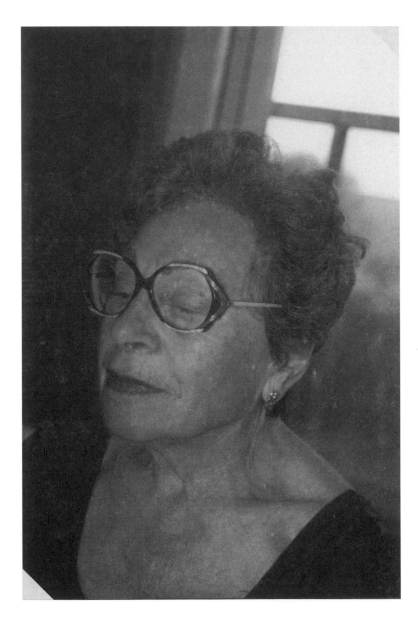

Covering the eyes to relax them

- Cup your hands a little and place them on your temples, over your eyes.
- Breathe deeply and calmly for a few minutes.

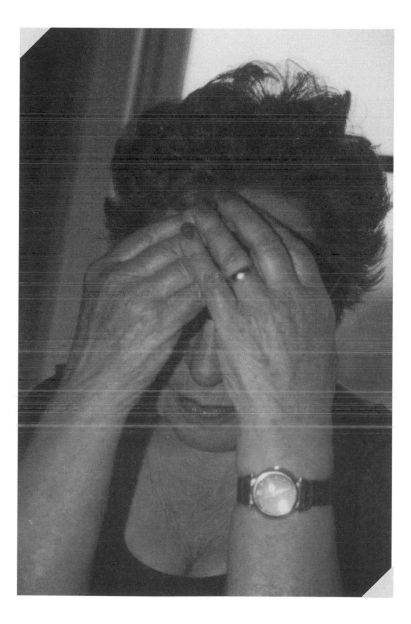

Energy (the force of vitality)

Fill yourself with energy!

This exercise can be performed standing, sitting or lying down.

- Place your hands loosely on your thighs, as follows:
- Your hands face upward, and are open to receive...
- Take a deep abdominal breath through your nose.
- Try to merge with the energy in your surroundings:

With your mind's eye, visualize green fields; make the color green flow to the weak organs in your body.

- Calm down and relax all your organs. Empty your mind of all thoughts for a few minutes.

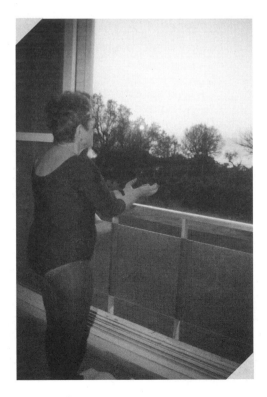

- Imagine that you are drawing strength from the sea and the sky, from the vegetation (flowers, bushes, lawns, and green trees).

- Draw strength from the dewdrops on the flowers.

- All this vitality penetrates your body.

- At this stage, your hands are red - they are receiving energy.

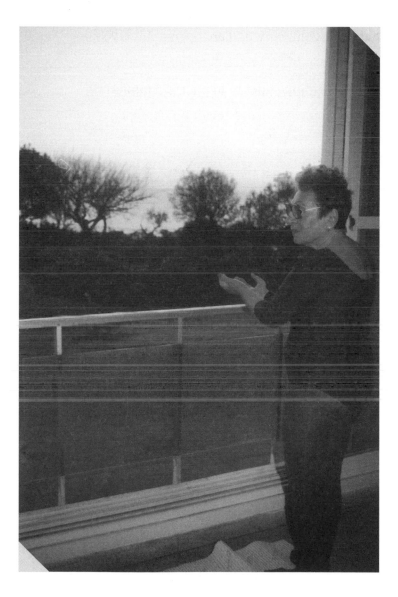

- Bring your hands close to your body:

- Place your hands on your head, on your neck, on your shoulders, and on all the rest of your organs.

- Breathe deeply and fill up with energy once more.

- Relax, and release all the tension.

- Place your hands on your chin.
  Your fingers face your ears, and your thumbs are below your lower jaw.

- Remain in this position for a few minutes, and say to yourself:
  "We will love ourselves, we will take care of ourselves!"

- Imagine that you are putting energy into the back of your head.
  Afterwards, place your hands behind your head.

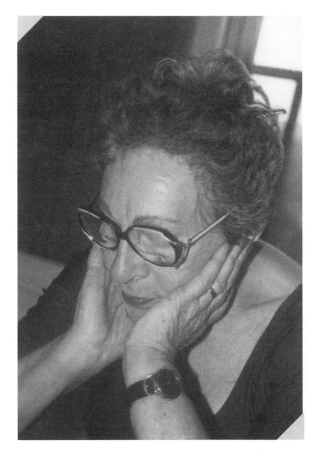

- Caress your body at a distance of five cm from it, hug yourself, and say:

  "I love myself."

  "I am very special."

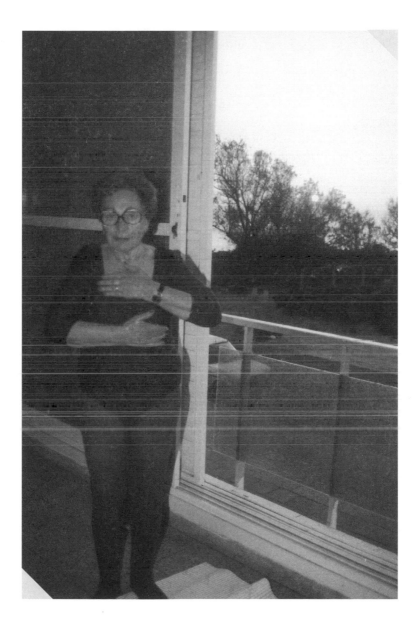

- Let energy penetrate your abdomen as follows:

  Place one hand above your navel.

  Place the other below your navel.

Do not cover your navel.

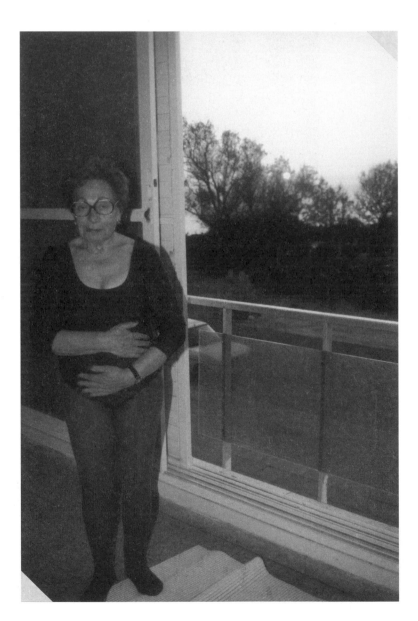

- Let energy penetrate your legs via your toes.
- Lift your feet a bit in the direction of your hands.
- Fill up with energy.

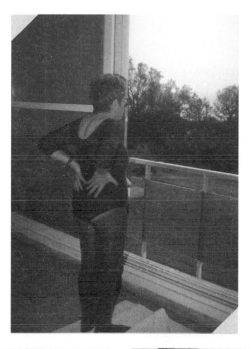

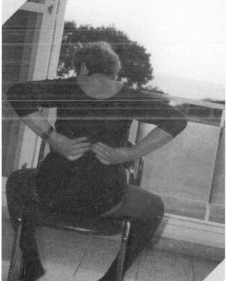
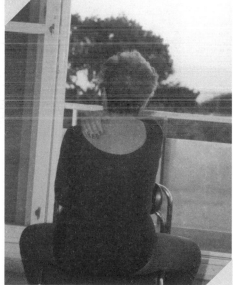

At all times in life,

especially during the hard times,

you must look at the bright side of life,

at the half-full glass.

Always think positively!

Let's try to accept ourselves as we are.

Exercises with chairs - standing

Positions for starting yoga exercises with chairs

– Standing facing the back of the chair.

– Standing with your back to the back of the chair.

– Standing in step position behind the back of the chair - so that the back of the chair is to the right of your body; holding the left side of the back of the chair with your right hand.

– Standing sideways beside the back of the chair beyond the end of the chair - so that the back of the chair is to the right of your body; holding the right corner of the back of the chair with your right hand, and the left corner with your left hand. Standing with your legs together beyond the legs of the chair.

Preparing your body

- Breathing: Inhale and exhale through your nose.
- Place the chair about a meter in front of you.
- Stand erect behind the chair, opposite its back.
- Lift your arms and stretch your body upward, breathing deeply.
- Bend the upper part of your body forward while exhaling.
- With two hands, grasp the back of the chair (inhale).
- Move your feet slightly backward. This stretches your back.
- Bend your knees.
- Let go of the back of the chair (exhale).
- Let your arms swing forward and backward.
  The upper part of your body is bent over.

This exercise helps release all the tension in the body.

Releasing the shoulder-blades

- Stand erect, your hands at your sides (inhale).
- Lift your shoulders.
- Move your shoulder-blades toward each other.
- Once more, bend the upper part of your body forward.
- Grasp the back of the chair with two hands.
- Stretch your buttocks backward (exhale).

In this exercise, your spine is stretched.

- Bend your knees.

Diagonal stretch

- Stand erect.
- Inhale and bend the upper part of your body forward.
- Hold onto the back of the chair with your right hand.
- Stretch your left arm forward and your right leg backward (exhale).
- Remain in this position for the count of 10.
- Relax.

Do this exercise three times.

Repeat this exercise on the other side:

- Inhale and bend the upper part of your body forward.
- Hold onto the back of the chair with your left hand.
- Stretch your right arm forward and your left leg backward (exhale).
- Remain in this position for the count of 10.

Do this exercise three times.

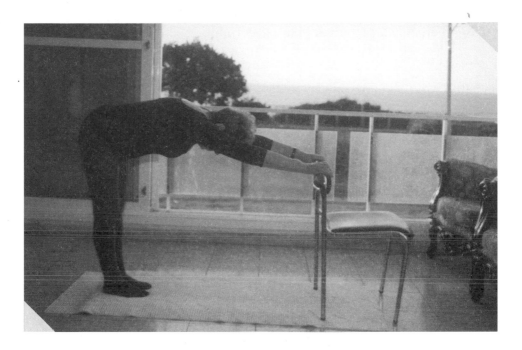

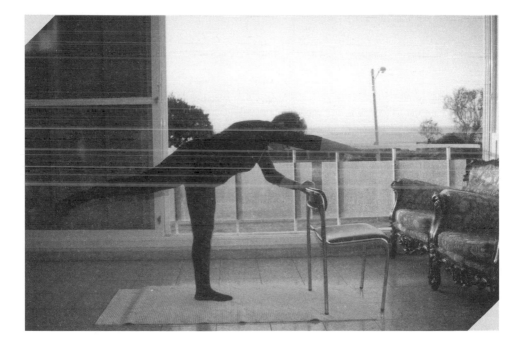

Leg seesaw for treating the thigh joints

- Stand erect at a distance of about 40 cm from the back of the chair.

- Hold onto the back of the chair with both hands.

- Inhale and stand on tiptoe.

- Lift your right leg as high as possible to the right, and take it over to the left in front of your body in a quick, flowing movement (exhale).

Do this movement 10 times.

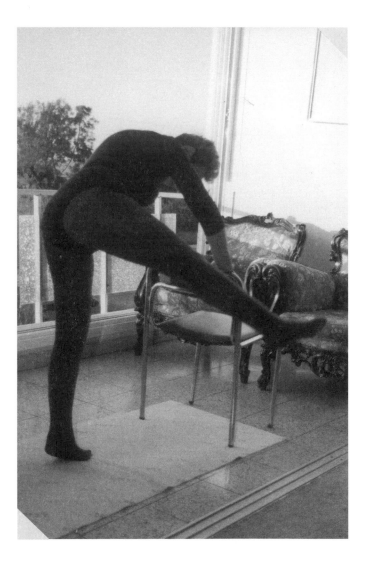

Repeat this movement with the left leg:

- Inhale and lift your left leg as high as possible to the left, and take it over to the right in front of your body in a quick, flowing movement (exhale).

Do this movement 10 times.

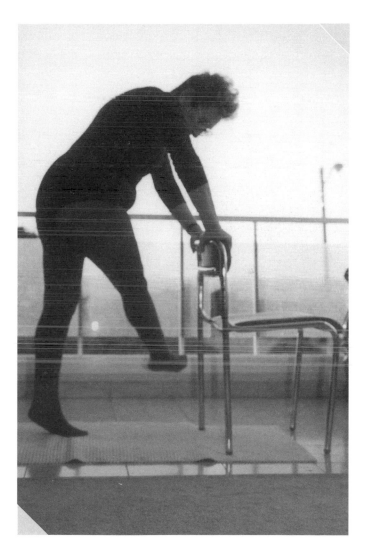

Exercises for the pelvis

Stage 1

- Stand erect (inhale).

- Stand on tiptoe.

- Hold onto the back of the chair with two hands.

- Stretch your right leg backward in the air.
  Your leg is in a straight line with your back (exhale).

- Remain in this position for the count of three.

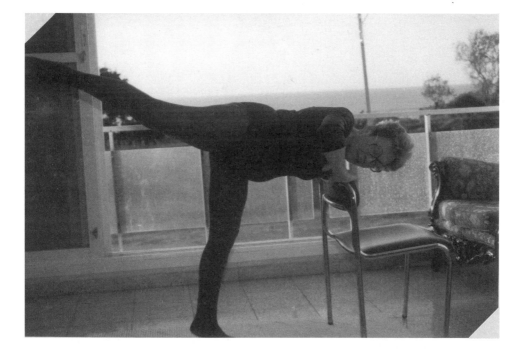

Stage 2

- Inhale and move your stretched right leg to the right at a 90-degree angle to your body (exhale).

- Remain in this position for the count of three.

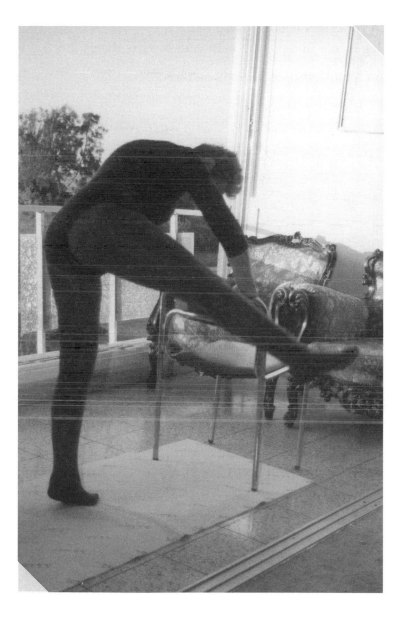

Stage 3

- Inhale and cross your right leg over your left leg.
- Remain in this position for the count of three (exhale).

Repeat this exercise with the left leg:

- Stand erect.
- Inhale and stand on tiptoe.
- Hold onto the back of the chair with two hands.
- Stretch your left leg backward in the air.
  Your leg is in a straight line with your back (exhale).
- Remain in this position for the count of three (inhale).
- Move your stretched left leg to the left at a 90-degree angle to your body (exhale).
- Remain in this position for the count of three.
- Inhale and cross your left leg over your right leg.
- Remain in this position for the count of three (exhale).

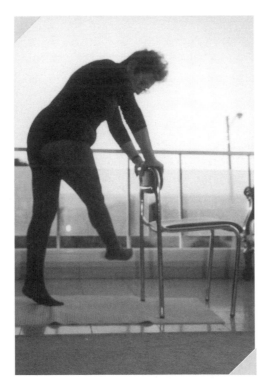

Releasing the pelvis

- Stand erect.

- Hold onto the back of the chair with two hands.

- Stand on tiptoe (inhale).

- Bend your right knee slightly.

- Turn your right knee inward and outward in as big turns as possible, clockwise and then anti-clockwise (exhale).

- Move your leg to the left, and then straighten it on the floor. Move your leg to the right and straighten it on the floor.

Do this exercise five times with the right leg.

Repeat the exercise with the left leg:

- Stand erect.

- Hold onto the back of the chair with two hands.

- Stand on tiptoe (inhale).

- Bend your left knee slightly.

- Turn your left knee inward and outward in as big turns as possible, clockwise and then anti-clockwise (exhale).

- Move your leg to the right, and then straighten it on the floor. Move your leg to the left and straighten it on the floor.

Do this exercise five times with the left leg.

Strengthening the back

Right side

- Stand erect.

- Hold onto the back of the chair with two hands (inhale).

- Lift your right knee and move it close to your nose.
  Your spine curves.

- Stretch your leg backward.
  Your knee is slightly bent, your heel faces the ceiling.
  Your spine straightens out.

- Remain in this position for the count of five.

- Relax (exhale).

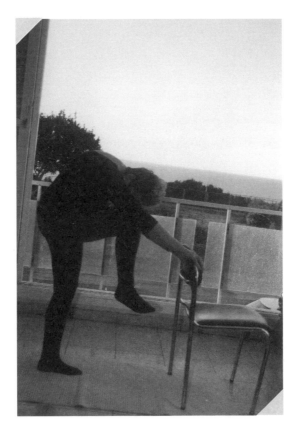

Left side

- Stand erect.

- Hold onto the back of the chair with two hands (inhale).

- Lift your left knee and move it close to your nose.
  Your spine curves.

- Stretch your leg backward.
  Your knee is slightly bent, your heel faces the ceiling.
  Your spine straightens out.

- Remain in this position for the count of five.

- Relax (exhale).

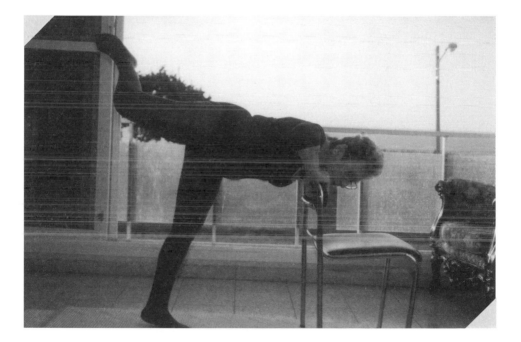

Leg twists

Right leg

- Stand erect.
- Stand on tiptoe.
- Hold onto the back of the chair with two hands (inhale).
- Lift your right leg, knee bent.
- Turn your knee from the thigh joint inward - to the left, and outward - to the right (exhale).

Do this exercise five times.

Left leg

- Stand erect.
- Stand on tiptoe.
- Hold onto the back of the chair with two hands (inhale).
- Lift your left leg, knee bent.
- Turn your knee from the thigh joint inward - to the right, and outward - to the left (exhale).

Do this exercise five times.

Stretching the side of the body

Right side

- Stand erect.

- Inhale and stretch your arms upward.

- Hold the center of the back of the chair with your left hand.

- Lift your right leg and your right arm.

- Stretch your arm and your leg.
  Your foot is stretched backward in a ballet position.
  Your arm goes forward, in line with the rest of your body.

- Relax while exhaling.

Do this exercise five times.

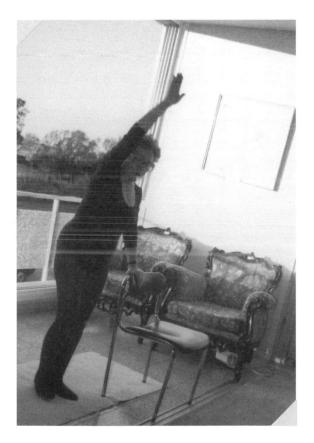

Left side

- Stand erect.

- Inhale and stretch your arms upward.

- Hold the center of the back of the chair with your right hand. Lift your left leg and your left arm.

- Stretch your arm and your leg.
  Your foot is stretched backward in a ballet position.
  Your arm goes forward, in line with the rest of your body.

- Relax while exhaling.

Do this exercise five times.

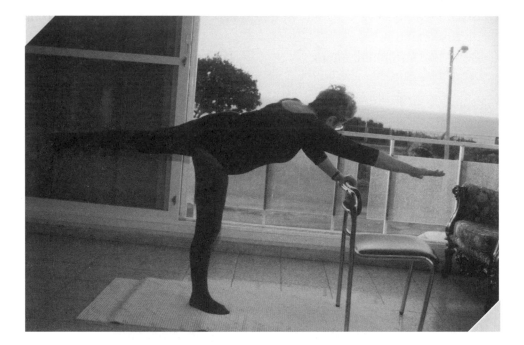

Releasing the shoulder-blades

- Come close to the chair and turn your back to it.
- Stretch your arms out behind, and grasp the back of the chair (inhale).
- Bring your shoulder-blades close together.
- Remain in this position for the count of five.
- Relax and contract again and then relax again.

Do this exercise three times.

Diagonal stretch

Stretching to the right

Your back is still turned to the back of the chair.
- Stretch your right hand backward and grasp the back of the chair (inhale).
- Lift your right leg, and grasp the outer side of your right foot with your left hand.
- Straighten your right leg and your left hand, which is holding it, in front of you (exhale).
- Bend and straighten again.

Do this exercise three times.

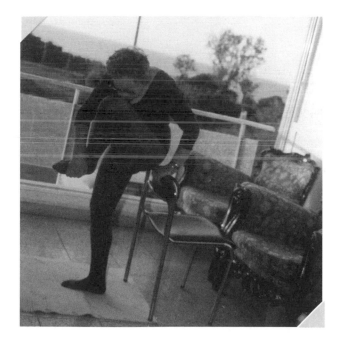

Stretching to the left

- Stretch your left hand backward and grasp the back of the chair (inhale).
- Lift your left leg, and grasp the outer side of your left foot with your right hand.
- Straighten your left leg and your right hand, which is holding it, in front of you (exhale).
- Bend and straighten again.

Do this exercise three times.

- Your back is still turned to the back of the chair.
- Hold onto the back of the chair with two hands, and bring your shoulder-blades close to each other by contracting them.

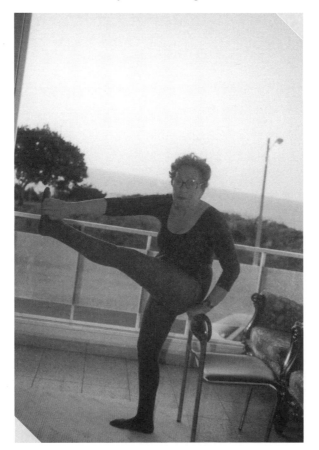

Stretching and balancing

Stretching to the right

- Stand so that the back of the chair is to the right of your body.

- Hold the back of the chair with your right hand (inhale).

- Stretch your left arm forward and your left leg backward.

- Move your left leg forward with impetus, and grasp your toes with your left hand.

- Stretch your left leg and your left hand, which is holding it, forward (exhale).

- Remain in this position for the count of three.

- Gently place your left leg on the floor.

Do this exercise three times.

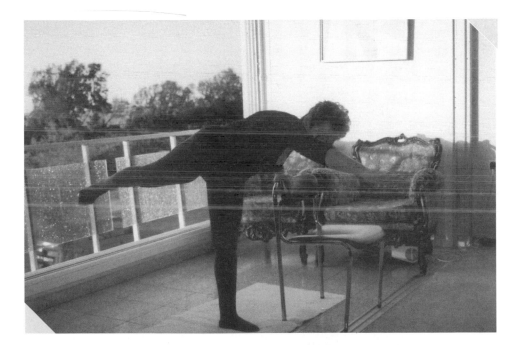

Stretching to the left

- Turn to the other side. Stand so that the back of the chair is to the left of your body.
- Hold the back of the chair with your left hand (inhale).
- Stretch your right arm forward and your right leg backward.
- Move your right leg forward with impetus, and grasp your toes with your right hand.
- Stretch your right leg and your right hand, which is holding it, forward (exhale).
- Remain in this position for the count of three.
- Gently place your right leg on the floor.

Do this exercise three times.

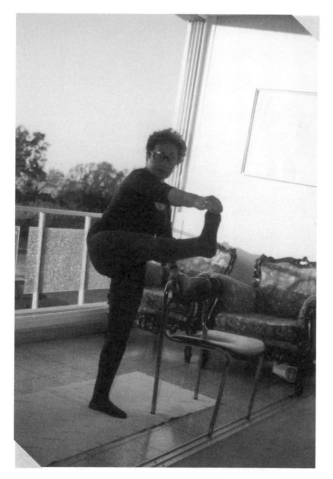

Releasing the sciatic nerve

Stage 1

- Stand next to the chair so that the left side of your body is close to the back of the chair.

  Your body does not face the back of the chair, but is turned to the right.

- Hold the left corner of the back of the chair with your left hand.

- Hold the right corner of the back of the chair with your right hand.

- Stand with your legs close together beyond the legs of the chair. Slowly bend your knees, and then straighten up.

Do this exercise 10 times.

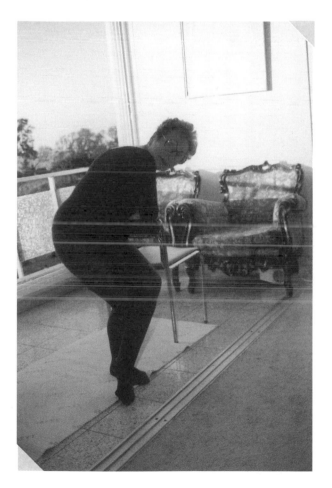

Stage 2

- Stand erect. Your hands remain in the same place (inhale).

- Cross your left leg behind your right leg.
  Your hip nerve is stretched.

- Cross your left leg in front of your right leg.

Bend both knees 10 times (exhale).

This movement prevents inflammations of the sciatic nerve.

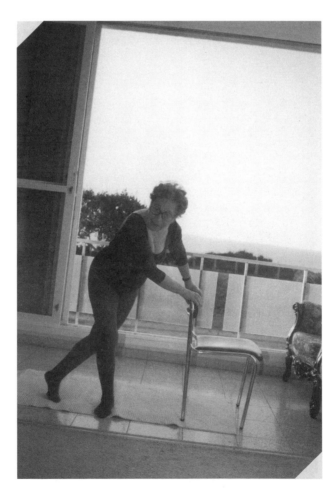

Stage 3

- Inhale and straighten your left leg backward in a maximum stretch at a 45-degree angle.
  Your right leg is slightly bent (exhale).

- Remain in this position for the count of 10.

- In this position, let your body sink slowly.
  Your left calf, the tendons and the nerves stretch and relax.

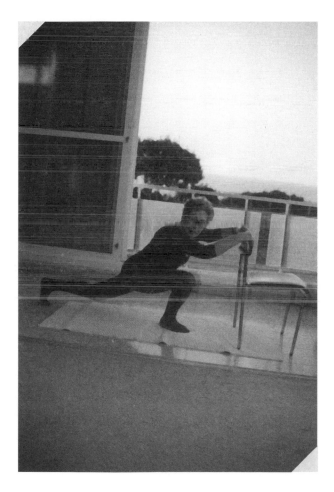

Repeat the exercise on the left side:

Stage 1

- Stand next to the chair so that the right side of your body is close to the back of the chair.
  Your body does not face the back of the chair, but is turned to the left.

- Hold the right corner of the back of the chair with your right hand. Hold the left corner of the back of the chair with your left hand.

- Stand with your legs close together beyond the legs of the chair.

- Slowly bend your knees, and then straighten up.

Do this exercise 10 times.

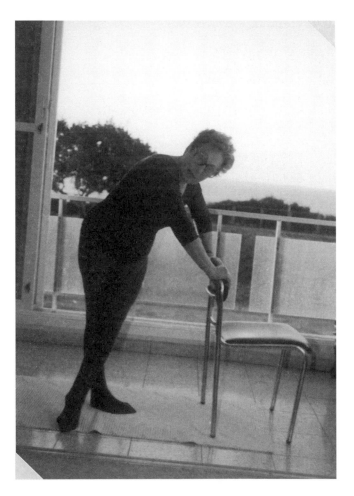

Stage 2

- Stand erect. Your hands remain in the same place (inhale).
- Cross your right leg behind your left leg. Your hip nerve is stretched.
- Cross your right leg in front of your left leg.

Bend both knees 10 times (exhale).

This movement prevents inflammations of the sciatic nerve.

Stage 3

- Inhale and straighten your right leg backward in a maximum stretch at a 45-degree angle.
  Your left leg is slightly bent (exhale).
- Remain in this position for the count of 10.
- In this position, let your body sink slowly.
- Your right calf, the tendons and the nerves stretch and relax.

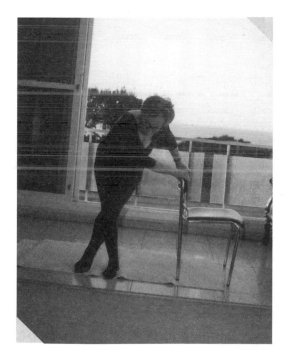

Treating the pelvis

- Stand so that the back of the chair is to the left of your body.

- Hold onto the back of the chair with your left hand.
  Your right hand rests on your hip (inhale).

- Lift your right leg and turn around so that you are facing the back of the chair.

- Bring your leg over the back of the chair.

- Place your foot on the seat.
  Your knee is bent at a 90-degree angle above the back of the chair (exhale).

- Take your foot down off the chair and place it on the floor in its place.

Do this exercise five times.

Repeat the exercise on the other side:

- Stand so that the back of the chair is to the right of your body.

- Hold onto the back of the chair with your right hand.
  Your left hand rests on your hip (inhale).

- Lift your left leg and turn around so that you are facing the back of the chair.

- Bring your leg over the back of the chair.

- Place your foot on the seat.
  Your knee is bent at a 90-degree angle above the back of the chair (exhale).

- Take your foot down off the chair and place it on the floor in its place.

Do this exercise five times.

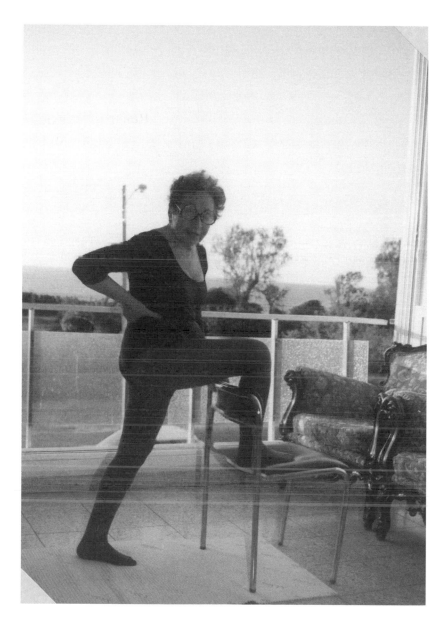

Stretching the spine

Right side

- Stand opposite the back of the chair (inhale).
- Lift your right leg over the back of the chair, and place your foot on the seat (exhale).
- Interlace your fingers behind you (inhale).
- Release your fingers.
- Stretch your arms upward, with the upper part of your body leaning forward (exhale).

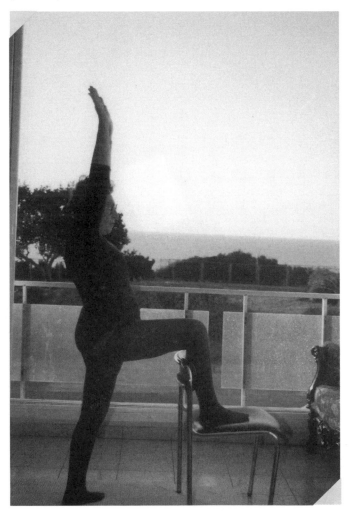

- Inhale and stretch your arms forward.
- Stand on tiptoe.
- Stretch your hands for a few seconds (exhale).
- Inhale and bend forward over the back of the chair.

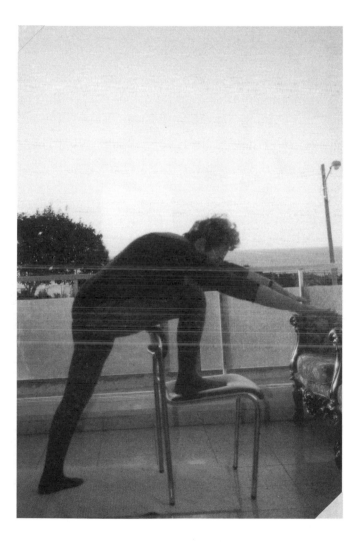

- Take hold of the front legs of the chair.

- Remain in this position for the count of three (exhale).

- Straighten up and relax your body.
  Your right foot is still on the chair.

Do this exercise five times.

- Take your right foot off the chair and place it on the floor.

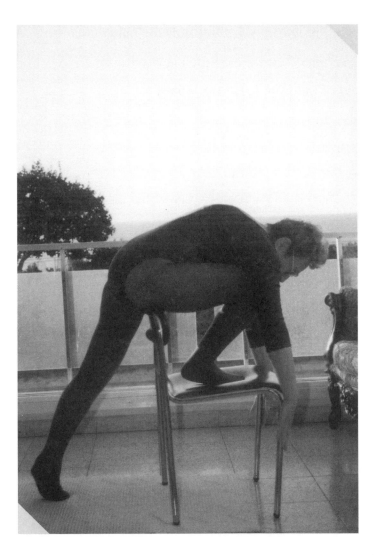

Left side

- Stand opposite the back of the chair (inhale).

- Lift your left leg over the back of the chair, and place your foot on the seat (exhale). Interlace your fingers behind you (inhale).

- Release your fingers.

- Stretch your arms upward, with the upper part of your body leaning forward (exhale). Inhale and stretch your arms forward.

- Stand on tiptoe.

- Stretch your hands for a few seconds (exhale).

- Inhale and bend forward over the back of the chair.

- Take hold of the front legs of the chair.

- Remain in this position for the count of three (exhale).

- Straighten up and relax your body.
  Your left foot is still on the chair.

Do this exercise five times.

- Take your left foot off the chair and place it on the floor.

Another powerful stretch of the entire body

Right side

- Stand erect (inhale).

- Lift your right leg and place your foot in the center of the back of the chair.

- Place your hands on the back of the chair on either side of your foot.

- Stretch your body backward in the direction of your buttocks for a few seconds.
  This stretches your entire body, as well as your leg and arms (exhale).

- Bring your nose close to your right knee, and your chest to your right thigh (inhale).

- Raise your left heel, and stand on tiptoe on your left foot.
  Your right knee is bent.

- Relax while exhaling.

Do this exercise three times.

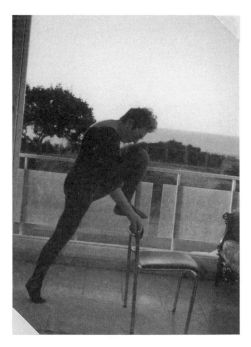
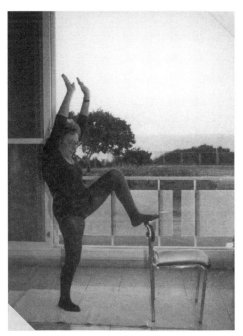

Left side

- Stand erect (inhale).

- Lift your left leg and place your foot in the center of the back of the chair.

- Place your hands on the back of the chair on either side of your foot.

- Stretch your body backward in the direction of your buttocks for a few seconds.

  This stretches your entire body, as well as your leg and arms (exhale).

- Bring your nose close to your left knee, and your chest to your left thigh (inhale).

- Raise your right heel, and stand on tiptoe on your right foot.
  Your left knee is bent.

- Relax while exhaling.

Do this exercise three times.

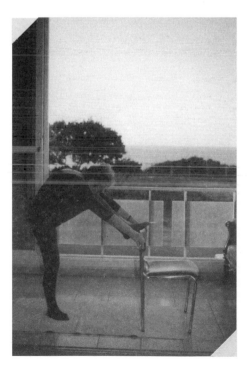
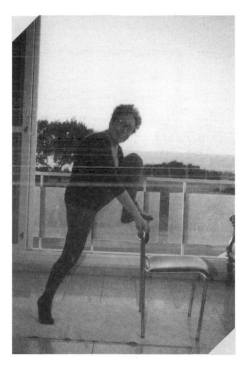

Bending forward

This exercise is done **without the chair**.
- Move away from the chair (inhale).
- Lift your arms up while standing erect.
- Bend the upper part of your body forward. Grasp your ankles with your hands: Your thumb faces forward, your fingers face backward. Your nose is close to your knees, and your chest rests on your thighs.
- Relax while exhaling.

Do this exercise three times.

Releasing the thighs
Turning the thighs like a clock

This exercise is done with the chair - stand behind the chair, opposite the back of the chair.

Right side

- Hold the back of the chair with your left hand (inhale).
- Place your straight right leg on the back of the chair.
- Hold the toes of your right foot in your right hand.
- Pull your right leg over the back of the chair, and then to the side, and then backward. Exhale throughout the movement.
  During the pulling, your standing leg swivels 45 degrees to the right and to the left.

Do this exercise three times.

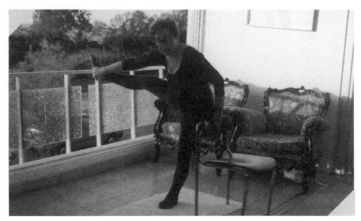

Left side

- Hold the back of the chair with your right hand (inhale).
- Place your straight left leg on the back of the chair.
- Hold the toes of your left foot in your left hand.
- Pull your left leg over the back of the chair, and then to the side, and then backward. Exhale throughout the movement.
  During the pulling, your standing leg swivels 45 degrees to the left and to the right.

Do this exercise three times.

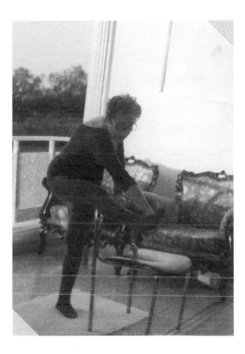

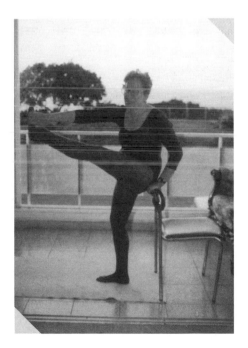

Exercise for effective kidney function

Right side

- Stand opposite the back of the chair.

- Hold the right edge of the back of the chair with your left hand.

- Turn to the right.
  Your left leg stands beside the right leg of the chair, the left side of your body is closer to the chair.

- Place your right leg behind your left leg, wide apart (step position).

- Turn to the left.

- Bend your left leg.
  Your left foot turns to the left in the direction of the chair.

- Inhale and lift your right arm.

- Pull your right arm over your head in the direction of the left corner of the back of the chair.

- Try to grasp the back of the chair.

- Remain in this position for the count of 10.

- Relax and straighten up while exhaling.

- Inhale and lift your left arm (which has been holding the right corner), and stretch it upward from the side and to the right.

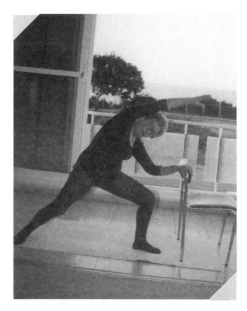

- While doing that, slide your right hand along your right leg for a side bend.

- Straighten up while exhaling.

Do this exercise three times.

Left side

- Stand opposite the back of the chair.
- Hold the left edge of the back of the chair with your right hand.
- Turn to the left.
  Your right leg stands beside the left leg of the chair, the right side of your body is closer to the chair.
- Place your left leg behind your right leg, wide apart (step position).
- Turn to the right.
- Bend your right leg.
  Your right foot turns to the left in the direction of the chair.
- Inhale and lift your left arm.
- Pull your left arm over your head in the direction of the right corner of the back of the chair.
- Try to grasp the back of the chair.
- Remain in this position for the count of 10.
- Relax and straighten up while exhaling.
- Inhale and lift your right arm (which was holding the left corner), and wave it upward from the side and to the left.
- While doing that, slide your left hand along your left leg for a side bend.
- Straighten up while exhaling.

Do this exercise three times.

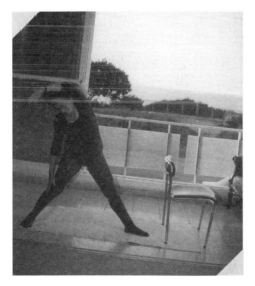 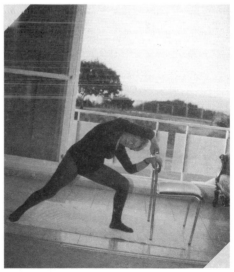

Exercises with chairs - sitting

Positions for starting exercises sitting on a chair

Sitting on a chair

– Sitting sideways:

Sit on the seat of the chair in such a way that one of the front corners is located between your spread legs.

– Regular sitting:

Your buttocks rest on the seat, and your back touches the back of the chair.

Exercises for sitting using chairs

Breathing: Inhale and exhale through your nose.

Stretching the side of the body

Right side

Stage 1

- Sit on a chair at a 45-degree angle.
  Your thighs are located on either side of the right corner of the seat.
  Your legs are spread.

- Grasp the seat with your left hand (inhale).

Stage 2

- Grasp your right foot in your right hand.

- Stretch it backward (knee bent) at the side of the seat.

- Remain in this position for the count of 10.

- Lift your right leg to your body.
  Your knee is very bent.

- Hold your right foot in your right hand.
  Your knee comes close to your stomach.

- Remain in this position for the count of 10.
  You feel the stretch in your outer thigh (exhale).

Stage 3

- Inhale and straighten your right leg and your right hand together (exhale).

- Stretch your leg upward.

- Remain in this position for a count of 10.
  Your tendons are stretched.

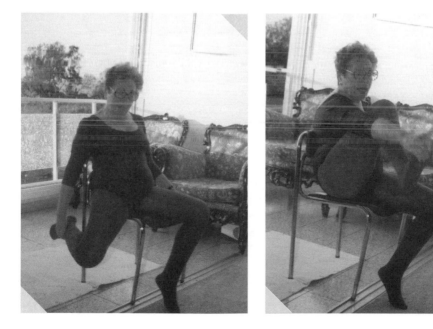

Stage 4

- Inhale and relax your arm and your leg.

- Stretch your right arm to the left and forward, and straighten your right leg behind you, at the side of the chair.
  Your toes touch the floor (exhale).

- Remain in this position for the count of 10.

Do this exercise three times.

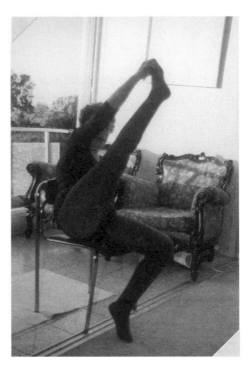

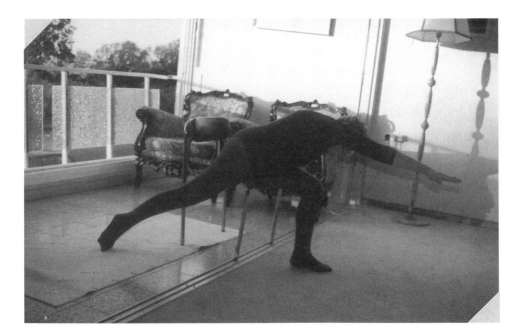

Left side

Stage 1

- Sit on a chair at a 45-degree angle.
  Your thighs are located on either side of the left corner of the seat.
  Your legs are spread.

- Grasp the seat with your right hand (inhale).

Stage 2

- Grasp your left foot in your left hand.

- Stretch it backward (knee bent) at the side of the seat.

- Remain in this position for the count of 10.

- Lift your left leg to your body.
  Your knee is very bent.

- Hold your left foot in your left hand.
  Your knee comes close to your stomach.

- Remain in this position for the count of 10.
  You feel the stretch in your outer thigh (exhale).

Stage 3

- Inhale and straighten your left leg and your left hand together (exhale).

- Stretch your leg upward.

- Remain in this position for the count of 10.
  Your tendons are stretched.

Stage 4

- Inhale and relax your arm and your leg.

- Stretch your left arm to the right and forward, and straighten your left leg behind you, at the side of the chair.
  Your toes touch the floor (exhale).

- Remain in this position for the count of 10.

Do this exercise three times.

Strengthening the thighs

- Sit on the chair with your legs apart.

- Place your hands on your thighs next to your groin.

- Inhale.

- Try to press your thighs together. (Your hands try to push your thighs apart.)

- Relax while exhaling.

Do this exercise five times.

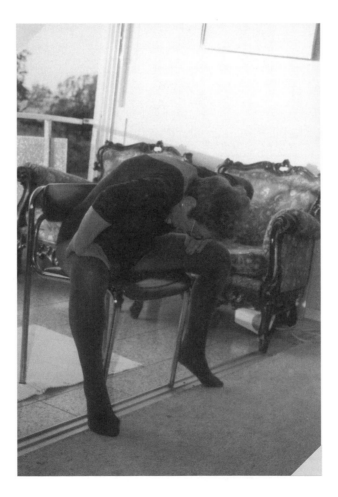

The baby in the cradle exercise

This can also be done on the floor (as shown in the photo).

- Sit on the chair with legs apart (inhale).

Right leg

- Lift your right leg.

- Grasp your right foot, and place it in the inner elbow of your left arm like a baby in a cradle.

- Rock your arms holding your foot left and right as if it were a baby.

- Relax and exhale.

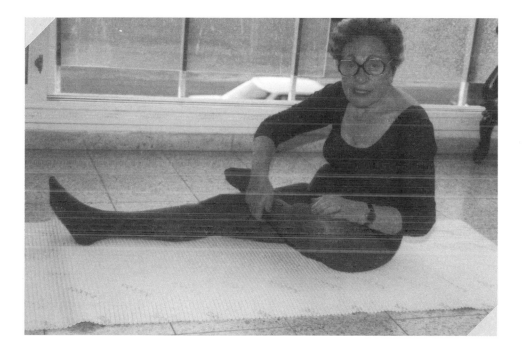

Left leg

- Inhale and grasp your left foot, and place it in the inner elbow of your right arm like a baby in a cradle.

- Rock your arms holding your foot right and left as if it were a baby.

- Relax and exhale.

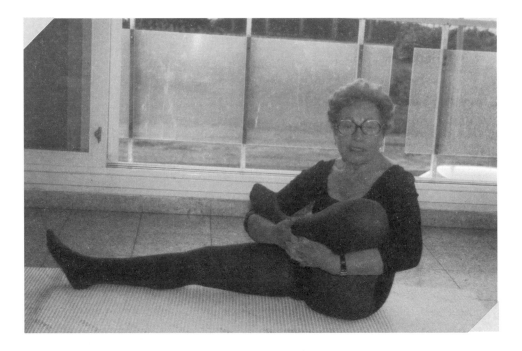

Stretching the shoulder-blades (1)

Right side

- Sit on the chair with your legs slightly apart.
- Inhale and place both hands below your right foot.
- Bring your right knee close to your nose, bending your leg.

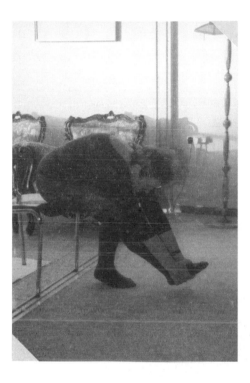

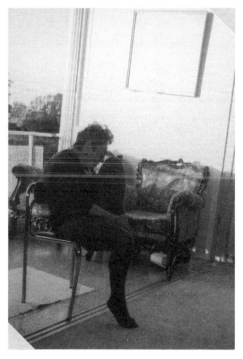

- Lift your foot and straighten it.

- Put it down slowly and gently (exhale).

- Feel the movement between the shoulder-blades.

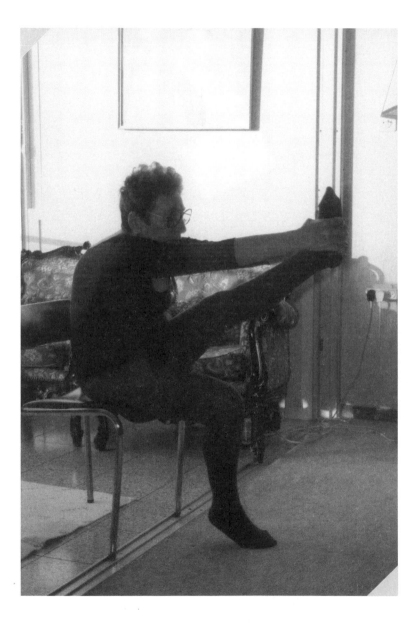

Left side

- Inhale and place both hands below your left foot.
- Lift your foot and straighten it.
- Put it down slowly and gently (exhale).
- Feel the movement between the shoulder-blades.

An additional option is to do the exercise on a mattress (as shown in the photo).

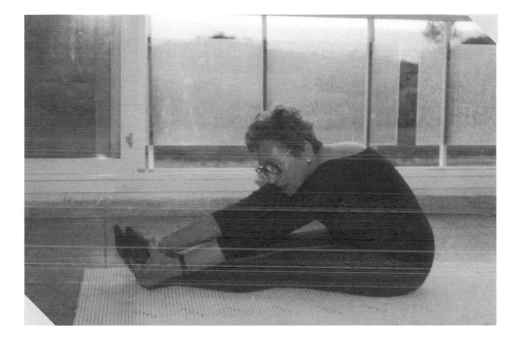

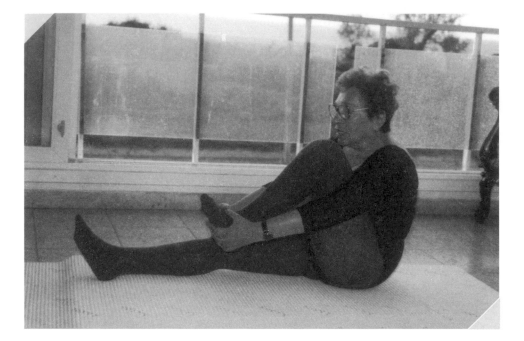

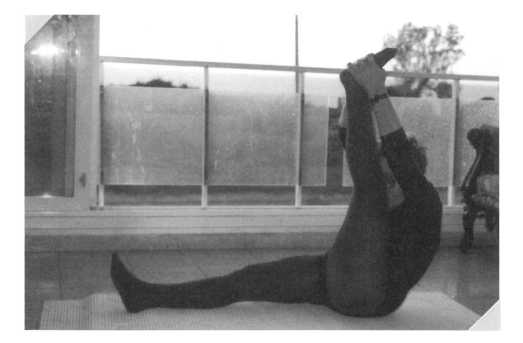

Stretching the shoulder-blades (2)

This exercise can also be done on a mattress (as shown in the photo).

Stage 1

- Sit on the chair and interlace your fingers behind the back of the chair.
- Pull your joined hands toward the floor.
- Move your shoulder-blades close to each other, and release.

Do this exercise three times.

Stage 2

- Sit relaxed on the chair and place your hands on your thighs, your curved palms facing upward (inhale).
- Turn your head toward your right shoulder, roll it onto your chest, raise it toward your left shoulder, and roll it backward (exhale).
- Inhale and turn your head to the right, looking over your right shoulder (exhale).
- Inhale and turn your head to the left, looking over your left shoulder (exhale).
- Inhale and bend your head onto your chest (inhale).
- Inhale and roll your head backward carefully (exhale).
- Place your hands on your hips (inhale).
- Bend your whole body to the right at the waist and straighten up (exhale).
- Inhale and bend your whole body to the left at the waist and straighten up (exhale).
- Inhale and turn your head around clockwise in a big, slow circle five times (exhale).
- Inhale and turn your head around anti-clockwise in a big, slow circle five times.
- Exhale and relax.
- Inhale and place both your hands below your right foot.
- Lift your leg and straighten it. Put it down gently and slowly (exhale). You can feel the movement between your shoulder-blades.

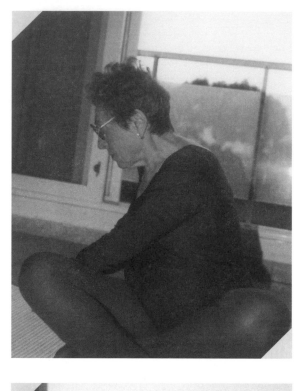

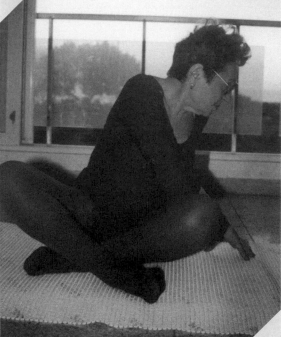

Advice for maintaining good health

Health Tips

● Good and useful advice

Every day is tomorrow's yesterday.

Therefore, look after yourself today so that you will be healthy tomorrow.

● Diet

Eat food that contains fiber - whole-wheat bread, brown rice, legumes!

Season with medicinal herbs.

Eat food that does not contain food coloring and preservatives!

● Physical exercise

The yoga method is effective for the whole body, including the internal organs.

● Sleep and relaxation

Ten minutes' relaxation is the equivalent of two hours' sleep during the day.

One hour of sleep before midnight is the equivalent of four hours' sleep after midnight.

What pupils say - personal stories

It's a great honor for me to say a few words about Rosie.

For me, she's a light in the darkness.

I always enjoy meeting her and her wonderful smile.

The yoga she teaches immediately roused something in me that is right for me.

All the movements are "right" for me and develop all my human abilities: physical, emotional, and rational.

Since I have been studying kinesiology, it suits me and supplements yoga.

I hope that I will be able to go into these studies in depth because I like them and enjoy them very much.

Thanks to Rosie who, at her venerable age, enjoys sharing the treasure within her with everyone.

Yael

My love story with Rosie began a few years ago, and I am grateful for the opportunity that was given me. Knowing Rosie, her sense of humor and her joie de vivre, her worldview and her personal wisdom, have given me a new perspective on life.

I hope that this book will be a guide to many people who want to change their lives through yoga.

Through yoga, we attain better health and fulfillment.

Love, Zippi Ben-Ari

To my guide!

Yoga lessons with Rosie mean embarking upon a spiritual journey, linking up to the focal point of emotions, and finally emerging as another person, a person who is happier and more at one with himself. All this thanks to you, my wonderful teacher Rosie, whose name symbolizes what you are perfectly. Thank you again!

Daniela Koren

I have never stuck to anything or persevered as I have in my yoga lessons with Rosie. A yoga lesson with Rosie always begins with a warm, personal greeting, a broad smile on her face. Naturally, we sometimes got to the lesson tired or troubled. When we crossed Rosie's threshold, everything vanished, and smiles could be seen all around.

It wasn't only the yoga lessons that made us persevere with Rosie - after all, yoga is available everywhere. Rosie's personality and personal example - practicing what she preaches - were the secrets that won our hearts.

I have had the privilege of being her pupil for about 20 years. After the lesson, we would sometimes go out to a cafe to drink a mixture of natural juices and to chat. I know about Rosie's hard life. "Hard" is a euphemism. However, despite the suffering she has known in her life, she remembered and remembers only the periods of happiness. She is optimistic and joyful about every new day that dawns.

Rosie succeeds in instilling in her pupils her wise, healthy, and convincing way of thinking. By means of joy and humor and her belief that yoga is ageless, whoever does yoga is young.

To Rosie with endless love.

The Matos family, Even Yehuda.
Rivka.

Yoga with Rosie is a special experience.

The yoga lesson with Rosie is unique.

First, as soon as you enter, you receive Rosie's personal loving, warm greeting of peace.

The pale pink carpet is pleasant underfoot, and the sea that is visible beyond the green garden opposite the broad window is conducive to a lesson in a special and pleasant atmosphere. This is all complemented by Rosie's own landscapes that adorn the walls.

And, of course, the main thing - the lesson itself.

No lesson is identical to another - Rosie always adds and innovates and incorporates new yoga exercises. While doing the exercises, I really feel the energy flowing, especially in my hands.

Rosie is involved in the participants' specific problems and tries to conduct her lesson accordingly. Frequently, a problem is solved in just one lesson, sometimes in a few. I had a problem in the elbow, which was diagnosed as an inflammation. I suffered from terrible pain. Rosie diagnosed that several tendons had become dislocated, and treated me for a few minutes. Afterwards, during the lesson, she gave me exercises that were meant especially for the arms. While I had been unable to work beforehand, during the lesson my arm could function once more.

Every lesson with Rosie provides a good start to the next day. We leave the lesson smiling, full of energy, ready to face another long, good day.

Love,
Yael Wiener

Meeting Rosie is meeting a person with endless joie de vivre.

Rosie smiles at everyone and creates a pleasant atmosphere in a framework that suits her and her job like a glove - just like the sea combines perfectly with the green, blooming garden outside and with Rosie's paintings inside.

Rosie is an astounding person who has profound knowledge of the human body and the diagnosis of its problems.

It is so good and pleasant to be in her company and to participate in her yoga lessons. When we leave each lesson, it is as if we have been born again.

With love and gratitude,
Shoshana Wiener

Two years ago, I arrived at Rosie's apartment, and I haven't torn myself away since.

My life has changed as a result of meeting this special woman. Today, yoga is a part of my daily life.

Rosie radiates an abundance of light and harmony, which she shares with everyone.

In my opinion, her humility is one of her outstanding qualities, and I thank her for the seed she planted in me - which germinated.

Susan

I have been doing yoga for 18 years, and it is, in my opinion, the ultimate physical and mental exercise form. At the end of the lesson, my body no longer feels tired, my mind is alert, and a feeling of good health envelops me.

Three years ago, I underwent complicated surgery, and thanks to yoga, I succeeded in coping with it and coming out triumphant. The doctors agreed that the wonderful ability to breathe as well as the correct muscle mass afforded a speedier recovery.

My great luck is that my teacher and guide is Rosie. In my opinion, the teacher's place in the exercise is extremely important, and Rosie is very professional and responsible in her work.

The fact that she declares that yoga is not a "competition" and that a person must listen to his body means that the lessons can be an experience of friendship and openness. Her quiet and love affect the entire group.

The end of the lesson always provides optimism for facing the new day.

For me, yoga is life, health - those are Rosie's words and I believe in them completely.

Ruty Riv

I live in a village that is quite far from Rosie's apartment, making it difficult for me to get there twice a week for yoga lessons. However, from the moment I met her, I was attracted to her warmth, love, fierce desire to help, and abundant creativity in "inventing" new exercises for people who needed them.

At Rosie's place, I have met women and pupils who are prepared to lend a hand at any time, and with Rosie's help, to understand every movement and its importance - to body and mind.

I learned to consume natural food, and to think positively. I persevered for 10 years, until my illness. I believe that I succeeded in overcoming the severe health problem I had - thanks to the great amount of knowledge I acquired from Rosie.

Love,
Alta

Fran's story - how this book became a reality

I began to participate in Rosie's yoga lessons about four years ago. Even during very busy times, I tried to keep it up at least once a week. The perseverance and internalization enabled me to look positively at myself and my surroundings. I felt as if I was undergoing a process of change that became significant for my family as well.

My self-confidence increased.

My body became stable and pliant.

I felt elated in spirit and soul.

I ate correctly.

A window of opportunities opened up before me as a result of ever-increasing awareness.

My personal acquaintance with Rosie, her joie de vivre, her overflowing optimism, and the vitality she radiates sparked the idea that it is important to attempt to preserve and share this knowledge with others. As a result, while practicing, I began to write down the exercises.

Every lesson is rich and varied, and the exercises in this book are just a portion of Rosie's treasure trove of exercises that she has developed during her work and according to her pupils' needs.

Many thanks to my husband Danny and to my four children, who sometimes had to miss out on precious time with me and forego the computer so that I could compile this book.

Thanks to my friends who encouraged me.

It is my hope that this book will bring you health, and will open up a better world for you and an understanding of your body and of other people.

Fran Naim